Abdellatif Maamri
Inass Hamdi
Souad Ben El Mostafa

Type 2 diabetes and high blood pressure

Abdellatif Maamri
Inass Hamdi
Souad Ben El Mostafa

Type 2 diabetes and high blood pressure

Risk factors in a population of women in the city of Berkane

ScienciaScripts

Imprint

Any brand names and product names mentioned in this book are subject to trademark, brand or patent protection and are trademarks or registered trademarks of their respective holders. The use of brand names, product names, common names, trade names, product descriptions etc. even without a particular marking in this work is in no way to be construed to mean that such names may be regarded as unrestricted in respect of trademark and brand protection legislation and could thus be used by anyone.

Cover image: www.ingimage.com

This book is a translation from the original published under ISBN 978-620-3-45345-4.

Publisher:
Sciencia Scripts
is a trademark of
Dodo Books Indian Ocean Ltd. and OmniScriptum S.R.L publishing group

120 High Road, East Finchley, London, N2 9ED, United Kingdom
Str. Armeneasca 28/1, office 1, Chisinau MD-2012, Republic of Moldova, Europe
Printed at: see last page
ISBN: 978-620-5-90591-3

Type 2 Diabetes and Arterial Hypertension: Risk Factors in a Population of Women in the City of Berkane

Table of contents

Summary:

Introduction: Diabetes, especially type 2, and hypertension as chronic diseases are major public health problems worldwide.

This work allows us to describe and analyse the most frequent risk factors associated with these pathologies, as well as the possible relationships between them.

Methods: We conducted an epidemiological, cross-sectional, descriptive and analytical study among 150 women aged 18 to 85 years, residents of the city of Berkane. The results presented in this work are based on data collected from a questionnaire containing sociodemographic, anthropometric and biological characteristics, which were processed and analysed using XLSTAT software.

Results: Our study population had a mean age of 50.3 years (standard deviation = 12.02 years), BMI of 30.36 kg.m-2 (±7.3), the incidence of diabetes was 25% with only 45% of diabetics being on treatment, and 24% having a balanced hba1c. The incidence of overall hypertension was 54% with 39% of the hypertensives undergoing treatment for hypertension. Multivariate analysis showed significant associations ($P<0.05$) between the occurrence of these two diseases and several risk factors, notably: age, obesity, abdominal obesity and hypercholesterolemia. These results are in agreement with several national and international studies.

Conclusion: In order to target prevention actions for these two chronic diseases and their complications and their early management, a better knowledge of women's lifestyle and eating and sports habits must be developed through the surveillance and monitoring system, as well as particular attention to the age of these diseases and the interest of prevention at an early age.

Key words: type 2 diabetes, hypertension, risk factors, complications, chronic diseases.

Introduction :

The chronic disease epidemic is affecting both developed and developing countries, and is linked to changes in diet and lifestyle (WHO & FAO, 2003). The burden of these chronic diseases is rapidly increasing worldwide. According to the World Health Organisation (WHO), these diseases kill 41 million people each year, accounting for 71% of deaths worldwide (WHO & FAO, 2003) more than all other causes of death. In low- and middle-income countries, the burden remains heavy: 78% of deaths are due to non-communicable diseases with 85% of premature deaths (Maamri & Ben El Mostafa, 2020).

Most countries in the world are experiencing changes in diet and behaviour, particularly in foods that are higher in fat and energy and lifestyles that are more sedentary - this change is driven by increasing industrialisation, urbanisation and mechanisation (WHO, 2002). Chronic diseases caused by diet include diabetes mellitus, obesity, cardiovascular disease, stroke, hypertension and certain types of cancer (WHO & FAO, 2003).

The more abrupt the lifestyle changes leading to obesity and sedentary lifestyle, the faster the incidence of type 2 diabetes and hypertension increases. WHO predicts that diabetes will be the seventh leading cause of death by 2030 (Abdelhay, 2017). Over the past decade, the incidence of diabetes has increased more rapidly in low- and middle-income countries than in high-income countries (WHO, 2016).

Similarly, hypertension is a very prevalent condition worldwide, in both developed and developing countries. The WHO has considered that the ageing of the population and rapid urbanisation are major contributors to the increased incidence of hypertension in urban areas (WHO EMRO, 2013).

The negative health consequences of high blood pressure are further compounded by the fact that many of the people affected also have other risk factors that increase their likelihood of suffering a heart attack, stroke or kidney failure. These risk factors include smoking, obesity, high cholesterol and diabetes mellitus (WHO, 2013).

NCDs are incurable and can cause various complications if not treated effectively. The aim of this work is to study the risk factors of diabetes and hypertension in a population of women in Eastern Morocco. Through the measurement and analysis of some socio-demographic, anthropometric and biological parameters.

I. Issue :

I.1 Magnitude and severity :

Since the 1990s, changes in diet and lifestyle have accelerated. As a result, chronic diseases such as diabetes and hypertension are becoming increasingly important causes of death. Today, almost 400 million people in the world suffer from diabetes with almost 4 million deaths each year (Belhadj *et al.*, 2019)and more than 1 billion people are hypertensive with 8.4 million deaths per year (WHO, 2013b).

In Morocco, these two types of chronic diseases constitute a major public health problem, given their exponentially increasing frequency. Today the frequency of diabetes in the adult population is more than 10.6% higher than that recorded in 2010 (6.6%) (Belhadj *et al.*, 2019). Between 2011 and 2018 the number of diabetics increased from 1.5 million to over 2 million (FZ *et al.*, 2018). The overall incidence of hypertension varies from 25 to 40% depending on the country and population considered. In 2000, it was 33.6%, 30.2% in men and 37% in women for a population aged 20 and over (Ministry of Health, 2000). These two pathologies are very dangerous, constitute an important cause of mortality and multiple complications. In 2003, hypertension was responsible for 5.9% of deaths, including 3.5% of women and 2.4% of men, and diabetes causes more than 24,000 deaths per year (Chraibi *et al.* 2012). This shows that we are facing a serious health problem.

I.2 Frequencies:

Morocco is undergoing considerable demographic and epidemiological transitions. The epidemiological and demographic transition is generally accompanied by a change in lifestyle, including dietary patterns and physical activity, and results in an increase in the burden of disease and mortality of NCDs, according to WHO these diseases are the leading cause of mortality with 80% of deaths in 2018, which places Morocco among the countries with high mortality from NCDs in the EMRO region (Ministry of Health, 2018).

This dietary transition from a traditional, cereal- and legume-based diet to one that includes more animal products tends to become excessive in relation to the energy needs of a sedentary life (Ministry of Health, 2011) .

According to the Ministry of Health, food consumption in Morocco has seen an overall increase in energy intake from 2202 Kcal in 1970 to 3031 Kcal in 2001 in urban areas, with strong disparities between urban and rural areas and between the richest and poorest (Ministry of Health, 2011) .

The phenomenon of overweight and obesity has increased significantly in Moroccan society. It is related to changes in diets and lifestyles, the origin of the epidemiological transition (Ministry of Health, 2011) . The frequency of diabetes and hypertension is increasing in parallel with obesity and lifestyle development. According to the Ministry of Health, 2 million Moroccan adults are estimated to be diabetic (FZ *et al.* 2018) of which eighty percent of diabetes cases in Morocco are type 2, i.e. linked to obesity and lifestyle (Belhadj *et al.*, 2019) . Thus, according to the results of the 2000 prospective survey of the Ministry of Health, the overall incidence of hypertension was 33.6%. With almost the same rate in the Arab countries around the Mediterranean (Chraibi *et al.* 2012) .

II. Literature review :

II.1 Definition of concepts :

II.1.1 Diabetes :

II.1.1.1 Definition:

Diabetes is a metabolic disorder characterised by the presence of hyperglycaemia due to reduced insulin secretion or insulin action, or both (Punthakee *et al.*, 2018).

The World Health Organization (WHO) defines the term "diabetes" as a metabolic disorder of multiple etiology, characterised by chronic hyperglycaemia accompanied by disturbances in carbohydrate, lipid and protein metabolism due to disorders in insulin secretion and/or action (insulin resistance).

Diabetes is defined as an elevation of fasting blood glucose above 7 mmol/L (1.26 g/L). The clinical diagnosis of hyperglycaemia is made by measuring plasma glucose levels, measured either fasting and/or randomly at any time of the day and/or during an oral glucose load (Tenenbaum *et al.*, 2018).

The criteria proposed by the American Diabetes Association (ADA) and recognised by the WHO for diagnosing diabetes are

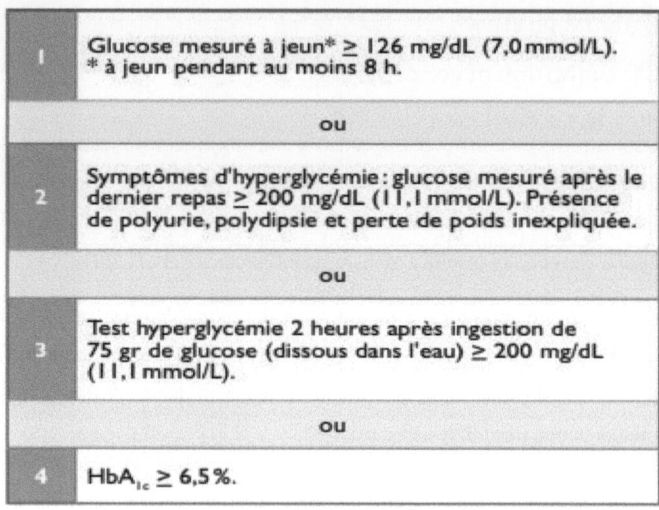

Figure 1 WHO diagnostic criteria (2006) (Tenenbaum *et al.*, 2018).

II.1.1.2 Classification:

Type 1 (formerly insulin-dependent) diabetes: Characterised by destruction of islet β-cells of autoimmune origin or unknown origin leading to absolute insulin deficiency, predisposing to ketoacidosis (Ministry of Health, 2016). Its onset is mainly in children or young adults. This type of diabetes represents less than 10% of diabetic patients (Bessire, 2000).

Type 2 diabetes (formerly non-insulin dependent diabetes mellitus (NIDDM)): Characterised by insulin resistance with or without a secretion defect. This type of diabetes appears in adulthood, and represents nearly 90% of diagnosed forms of diabetes (Bessire, 2000).

Gestational diabetes: Occurs during pregnancy (4-6% of pregnancies), usually towards the end of the second trimester and during the third. It is characterised by a normal decrease in insulin sensitivity which leads to an increase in the secretion of this molecule to maintain normal blood sugar levels (Ministry of Health, 2016).

Other types of diabetes: secondary to pancreatic pathology, genetic abnormality of β-cells or insulin receptors, related to an endocrinopathy, genetic syndrome, etc. (Bessire, 2000).

II.1.2 Obesity :

Obesity is the condition of an individual with a body mass significantly greater than is desirable or acceptable, usually due to an accumulation of body fat related to energy intake exceeding expenditure (Department of Health, 2016).

According to the WHO Overweight and obesity are defined as an abnormal or excessive accumulation of body fat that can impair health (WHO, 2003).

Obesity can be defined by the Body Mass Index (BMI), a simple index of weight for height commonly used for the classification of underweight, overweight and obesity in adults. It is calculated by dividing weight in kilograms by the square of height in metres (kg/m2) (WHO, 2003).

According to the WHO definitions, a distinction is made between :

Classes d'IMC	IMC (kg/m²)
Normale	18,5 à 24,9
Surpoids	25 à 29,9
Obésité modérée	30 à 34,5
Obésité sévère	35 à 39,9
Obésité trés sévère	supérieur à 40

Figure 2WHO BMI classification (WHO, 2013).

Obesity can also be defined by waist circumference measurement: Waist circumference >80 cm for women and >94 for men (WHO, 2013).

II.1.3 High blood pressure :

- **Blood pressure :**

Blood pressure is the force with which the heart pumps to send blood through the arteries and vessels, measured in millimetres of mercury (mm Hg). This gives two values, the first is the systolic blood pressure SBP (the highest pressure in the blood vessels) obtained when the heart is contracting and the second value is the diastolic blood pressure DBP (the lowest pressure in the blood vessels) obtained when the heart is relaxing (WHO, 2013b).

- **High blood pressure** :

High blood pressure, also known as high blood pressure. This is when the blood pressure in the arteries is permanently too high. It is dangerous, because it tires the heart, creates serious damage to the artery walls and causes cardiovascular accidents (The French Federation of Cardiology, 2019b).

High blood pressure is the leading cardiovascular risk factor, i.e. it greatly increases the risk of myocardial infarction, stroke, kidney failure, arteriopathy of the lower limbs... (The French Federation of Cardiology, 2019b).

AH has been defined according to WHO as a systolic blood pressure (SBP) $\geq$ 140 mmHg and/or a diastolic blood pressure (DBP) $\geq$ 90 mmHg, measured under standardised conditions at rest, in a sitting position, with a cuff adapted to the size of the subject's arm (WHO, 2013a).

II.1.4 Hypercholesterolemia :

Cholesterol :

It is an essential constituent of the cell wall, and is a component of many hormones and allows the synthesis of vitamin D. Of which 75% of cholesterol is produced by the liver and 25% by our diet (The French Federation of Cardiology, 2019a).

Cholesterol circulates in the blood using two types of transporters, cholesterol that goes from the cells to the liver and allows the elimination of cholesterol from the body ("good" cholesterol or HDL-cholesterol), and cholesterol that goes from the liver to the cells and is deposited on the walls of the arteries ("bad" cholesterol or LDL-cholesterol) (The French Federation of Cardiology, 2019a).

Hypercholesterolemia :

Hypercholesterolemia is the fact of having a blood level of cholesterol higher than normal. It can have a genetic origin, but also be linked to other diseases (hypothyroidism, diabetes...) (futura-sciences, 2018).

According to the French Federation of Cardiology, a total cholesterol level is "normal" when it is below 2g/L (French Federation of Cardiology, 2020).

II.2 State of knowledge :

II.2.1 Epidemiology of diabetes :

Diabetes is a widespread disease in the world with a high frequency, mainly type 2 diabetes which accounts for about 90% of all diabetics (Villar & Zaoui, 2010).

Worldwide, according to the WHO, 422 million adults were living with diabetes in 2014, compared to 108 million in 1980. This true epidemic was responsible for 1.5 million deaths in 2012, and 4 million deaths worldwide in 2017 (Belhadj *et al.*, 2019). Over the past decade, the incidence of diabetes has increased more rapidly in low- and middle-income countries than in high-income countries (WHO, 2016). It is one of the major diseases of the 19th century, responsible for 3.8 million deaths per year, which is similar in magnitude to deaths caused by the human immunodeficiency virus (HIV) (2.8 -3.5 million) (Arbouche, 2012).

In the Maghreb, the incidence of diabetes is higher. It is estimated at 9.8% in Tunisia for people aged 20-79 years in 2017, and at 14.4% in Algeria and 10.6% in Morocco for the population aged 18-79 years in 2018 (Belhadj *et al.*, 2019).

In Morocco, according to the Ministry of Health in 2018, more than 2 million people aged 18 years and over have diabetes, 50% of whom are unaware of their disease (FZ *et al.*, 2018). The frequency of diabetes in 2010 according to several studies was 6.6%, so according to the survey (2017-2018) in 2018 this frequency was 10.6%. (Belhadj *et al.*, 2019)and this figure will reach 2.5 million by 2030 (Shaw *et al.*, 2010).

II.2.2 Epidemiology of hypertension :

Hypertension, also known as high blood pressure, is one of the most serious and common health problems of our time.

Globally, the number of people with high blood pressure increased from 600 million to one billion between 1980 and 2008. The consequences of hypertension result in 8.4 million deaths per year, and this health problem is the direct cause of 13% of deaths worldwide. It is also the leading cause of 45% of cardiovascular deaths and 51% of stroke deaths. Therefore, hypertension is a global public health threat (WHO, 2013b). According to a study by a group of American and British researchers in 2000, based on data from 30 regional or national studies, 26.4% of adults had hypertension, for a total estimated number of 972 million people, 333 million in developed countries and 639 million in developing countries. Estimates for 2025 show that 29.2% of adults will be hypertensive (Kearney *et al.*, 2005).

In sub-Saharan Africa, this condition is on the rise. The ETHNA study carried out in North Africa in 2008 on a sample of 28,500 individuals found an incidence of hypertension of 41.8% in Algeria, 37.6% in Morocco and 20.6% in Tunisia (Nejjari *et al.*, 2013). Another study in Togo on hypertension and its risk factors conducted in May 2011 showed that the frequency of hypertension was 36.7%, including 34.6% of men and 38.4% of women (Yayehd *et al.*, 2013).

In Morocco, the frequency of hypertension is between 25 and 40% depending on the country and the population considered. According to a survey conducted by the Ministry of Health in 2000, the overall incidence of hypertension was 33.6%, 30.2% in men and 37% in women for a population aged 20 years and over (Ministry of Health, 2000)It decreased between 2000 (33.6%) and 2017 (29.3%) (Maamri & Ben El Mostafa, 2020). But despite this decrease, hypertension continues to cause enormous damage to health. In 2003, hypertension was responsible for 5.9% of deaths in Morocco, including 3.5% of women and 2.4% of men (Chraibi *et al.* 2012).

II.2.3 Risk factors for type 2 diabetes:

Obesity is the leading environmental risk factor for type 2 diabetes. The largest study that was done was that of Hu *et al* in 2001 on 84,941 nurses, which showed that having a BMI greater than 35 kg/m² multiplied the risk of diabetes by 20.1 (respectively by 28.8) in obese people (Hu *et al.*, 2001). The WHO recognises that a BMI of more than 25 kg/m2 puts an individual at risk of developing type 2 diabetes sooner or later (Hajar, 2016).

On the other hand, other studies have suggested that the location of fat at the trocar or a high waist to hip ratio (WHR) may also be a factor associated with the risk of diabetes (Grimaldi, 2004). Thus a 2007 meta-analysis by Vazquez *et al* confirmed that BMI, waist circumference, or WHR were associated with diabetes risk (Vazquez *et al.*, 2007).

Aging is indeed an important risk factor for type 2 diabetes due to both increased insulin resistance and reduced insulin secretion (Simon & Eschwege, 2002).

Many studies have established the association between **age** and type 2 diabetes as a risk factor. In fact, in the past the age of 45 years has been used as an important starting point for estimating the incidence of diabetes. Thus in recent years, young adults aged 30-39 years have experienced a surprising 70% increase in type 2 diabetes (Fletcher *et al.*, 2002).

High **blood pressure (BP) is an** important risk factor for mortality and disability, particularly in people with diabetes. People with high blood pressure have a greater risk of developing diabetes and people with diabetes also have an increased risk of high blood pressure. Several studies have investigated this association between T2DM and hypertension (Diyane *et al.*, 2013;Mengesha, 2007;DEMBELE *et al.*, 2000).

In addition, economic analyses have shown that strict BP control in diabetics is more cost-effective than strict blood glucose control (New *et al.*, 2003).

A sedentary lifestyle is a real public health problem. It significantly increases the risk of developing type 2 diabetes. Sedentary behaviour is described as "time spent in activities with low energy expenditure". This behaviour has been identified by several studies as a potential risk factor for diabetes and metabolic syndrome, independent of physical activity. A US study on the impact of sedentary behaviour on the development of diabetes in at-risk individuals found that the risk of developing diabetes increased by about 3.4% for every hour spent watching television (Rockette *et al.*, 2015).

According to another study, compared to those sitting <4 hours/day, participants reporting 4 to <6, 6 to <8 hours and ≥8 hours were significantly more likely to report ever having diabetes (George *et al.*, 2013).

While environmental factors are implicated in the development of diabetes, **genetics** may also play a role in the onset of the disease. Thus, the risk of becoming diabetic oneself if one of the parents is type 2 diabetic is about 35% and more if it is the mother rather than the father. And 70% if both parents are affected compared to about 10% in the general population (Philippe, 2014).

To estimate this relationship more precisely, studies are being carried out on monozygotic and dizygotic twins. Indeed, the probability that both twins have type 2 diabetes was at least twice as high in the case of monozygotic twins of about 70% (identical twins) compared to dizygotic twins of 20-30% (fraternal twins) (Philippe, 2014).

Other risk factors include lack of physical activity, a diet rich in trans fatty acids, smoking...

Several studies have shown that diabetes is linked to important risk factors, and we cite a few examples in this regard:

Table I Some work on diabetes and its risk factors.

Author	Target population	Sample	Website	Results
(Pan *et al.*, 1997)	The Chinese population.	Sample of 224,251 residents aged 25-64.	19 provinces and regions, including cities and rural areas in northern, southern, eastern and central China.	Diabetic subjects: -are older. -have an annual income higher personal costs. -are more likely to have a family history of diabetes. -a higher average BMI. -a higher waist to hip ratio (WHR). -systolic and diastolic blood pressure and a higher incidence of hypertension.
(Pan *et al.*, 1997)	The Chinese population.	Sample of 110,660 men and women from 33 clinics.	The city of Da-Qing in China.	-Diet is associated with a 31% (P<0.03) reduction in the risk of developing diabetes. -Exercise by 46% (P<0.005). -And exercise + diet by 42.1% (P<0.005). (In subjects with IGT).
(Tuomilehto *et al.*, 2001)		Sample of 522 subjects, 172 men and 350 women		-The risk of diabetes was reduced by 58% (P<0.001) by lifestyle change.

		with impaired glucose tolerance.		
(Balkau et al., 2008)		Sample of 1863 men and 1954 women aged 30-65 years.		significant differences in mean age P=0.0005, BMI P=0.0001, and incidence of hypertension P=0.02 between diabetics and non-diabetics.
(Benharra ts & Bencharif , 2019)	The Algerian populatio n.	A sample of 200 cases of schizophr enic patients hospitalis ed at the Sidi Chami psychiatri c hospital.	Oran, Algeria.	Among the risk factors for diabetes recorded by this study: age 40 and over, divorce, dyslipidaemia, high blood pressure, severe and moderate overweight and obesity, 30-40 years of schizophrenia, first generation antipsychotic treatment and family history of diabetes.
(Hu et al., 2001)		A sample of 84,941 female nurses.		-According to this study, body mass index is the most important risk factor for type 2 diabetes. -the relative risk of diabetes was 38.8 for women with a body mass index 35.0 or more and 20.1 for women with a body mass index of 30.0 to 34.9, compared to women with a body mass index of 30.0 to 34.9. who had a body mass index below 23.0.
(Musaige r & Al-Mannai, 2002)	The Bahraini populatio n.	Sample of 514 adults aged 30-79 years.	Bahrain.	-The overall incidence of diabetes was 9%. With a higher risk of diabetes in: older people (50-79 years), women, illiterate, currently married, non-smokers, those who did not walk regularly, overweight and obese (BMI> or = 25), those with a history of hypertension, and those who consumed fresh vegetables more than 3 times a week. -Only obesity was significantly associated with diabetes (OR = 1.83, CI 1.48-4.15).

(DEMBELE *et al.*, 2000)	Patients admitted to the Department of Internal Medicine.	Sample of 4848 patients.	The Internal Medicine Department of the Point G National Hospital - BAMAKO.	The frequency of the combination of hypertension and diabetes in this study was 16.7%. -This association was more frequent in women 21% (71/331) than in men 12% (41/340): P = 0,001. -It was more common from the age of 50 onwards.
(Mengesha, 2007)	The people of Gabon.	Sample of 401 patients.	Gaborone City Council (GCC) clinics. Gaborone, Botswana.	-In this study it was found that 61.2% of the patients with diabetes had high blood pressure, 56.4% had obesity, 33.5% had high cholesterol and 38.9% had high blood sugar. -Also hypertension was associated with age, sex, type of DM, body mass index (BMI) and hypertriglyceremia.
(Daousi *et al.*, 2006)	Urban population of 380,000 in the north of Liverpool, UK.	Sample of 3637 diabetic patients.	Liverpool, UK.	-In this study 86% of patients with type 2 diabetes were overweight or obese, 52% were obese and 8.1% were morbidly obese.
(Lotfi *et al.*, 2017)	Moroccan population.	Sample of 2227 diabetics (58% of women; 42% of men).	Kenitra, Morocco.	In this study, overweight affects the entire population. Pearson's correlation coefficients are highly significant (P<0.005) between BMI and fasting blood glucose (r = 0.5) and between BMI and glycosylated haemoglobin (r = 0.4).
(Diyane *et al.*, 2013)	Moroccan population.	100 hypertensive type 2 diabetic patients aged 65 years or older.	Marrakech, Morocco.	The sex ratio of the patients studied was 0.26, the mean age was 69.2 ± ; 4.3 years, the age of diabetes was 9.3 ± ; 6.7 years. Only 4.2% had an HbA1c ≤ 6.5%. The mean BMI was 28.1 ± 4.6 kg/m2. Dyslipidaemia was present in 59.6% of our patients, mainly hypoHDLaemia (75.9%).

Obesity is the main risk factor for diabetes, and several studies have shown that obesity is linked to several factors:

Table II Some work on obesity and its risk factors.

Author	Target population	Sample	Website	Results
(Janghorbani et al., 2007)	Iranian adults.	Sample of 89,404 men and women aged 15 to 65.	Iran.	In the course of this study -Age, low physical activity, low education, marriage and residence in urban areas were strongly associated with obesity. -Abdominal obesity was more common in women than in men (54.5% vs. 12.9%) and increased with age.
(Rahim & Baali, 2011)	A group of Moroccan women.	A sample of 343 (42.9%) Sahrawi women and 457 (57.1%) women from other ethnic groups in Morocco, aged between 20 and 62.	The city of Smara, Morocco.	-The percentage of obese women found is 43.5%. -Obesity is statistically associated with the biodemographic and socio-cultural indicators used in this study (age, level of education, perception of body image, geographical origin of women). -Geographical location in the Sahara or in other parts of Morocco appears to be the factor most associated with obesity.
(Rguibi & Belahsen, 2004)	Moroccan population.	Sample of 249 Sahrawi Moroccan women, aged 15 and over.	Sahara, Morocco	The results of this study indicate that central obesity was the most common comorbid factor (75%) (with a frequency of obesity of 49%) followed by hypertension (28.6%), hypertriglyceridaemia (22.4%), hyperglycaemia (11.9%) and hypercholesterolaemia (11.6%).
(Fafa et al., 2015)	The Algerian population.	2210 subjects (1583 women and 627 men) aged	Algiers (Algeria).	According to this study, the incidence of overall obesity was 24.9%. The incidence of android obesity was 66.4%. Multivariate analysis showed that age, female gender, low education level, family or

| | | 18-64 years. | | personal history of obesity and menopause were at risk of overall android obesity. While younger age, higher education, male gender, single status and high physical activity were at low risk of global and android obesity. |
| (Zhang *et al.*, 2008). | The Chinese. | 6643 people aged 60. | Fuxin County, Liaoning Province, China | According to the World Health Organization criteria, the results of this study show that the incidence of overweight and obesity was 13.8 and 1.7%, respectively. A positive association was also observed between body mass index and female gender, Mongolian nationality, education levels and current alcohol consumption. And an inverse association between body mass index and age, physical activity levels and current smoking. |

II.2.4 Risk factors for hypertension :

Non-modifiable factors :

There is a linear relationship between **age** and hypertension, as the characteristics of blood pressure change with age (sodium sensitivity, endothelial dysfunction...) (CAMBOU, 2010).

According to a survey carried out in 2007 (FLASHS) in 2002 the percentage of hypertensives varies according to age group, rising from 4.2% for those under 45 to 51.8% for those over 75. In 2007 it rose from 5% to 59% (Girerd & Murino, 2007). (Girerd & Murino, 2007). Moreover, many other studies have shown this relationship (Benharrats & Bencharif 2019;Musaiger & Al-Mannai 2002)....

Male gender has also been considered as a risk factor for hypertension, as men tend to become hypertensive earlier in life than women. This has been shown by several studies. According to the MONA LISA study, conducted between 2005 and 2007, hypertension was present in 47% of men and 35% of women, i.e. 23.9% and 8.4% respectively between the ages of 35-44 and 79.8% and 71.3% for those aged 65-75 (WAGNER *et al.*, 2008).

The **hereditary** nature of hypertension has been well established by numerous family and twin studies, which have estimated a clinical heritability of systolic and diastolic blood pressure of between 15-40% and 15-30% respectively (Feinleib *et al.*, 1977;Staessen *et al.*, 2003).

Modifiable factors:

Overweight and obesity are among the factors influencing the rise in blood pressure. The higher the body mass index (BMI), the higher the risk of hypertension...

Thus, several authors have shown that there is a close relationship between obesity and high blood pressure, especially android obesity (Sellam & Bour, 2016;Bruckert, 2008;Ginsberg & Maccallum, 2009). Indeed, the risk of hypertension is 3 times more frequent in obese subjects than in normo-weight people and obese people have an increased risk of hypertension compared to slim subjects (WHO, 2003).

Hypertension promotes the development of type 2 **diabetes** through various mechanisms. **Diabetes** is also recognised as a risk factor for the development of hypertension. About 80% of T2DM patients will eventually develop hypertension (Scheen *et al.*, 2012).

Smoking is also an important risk factor for hypertension. It has both short- and long-term adverse effects on the heart and blood vessels, and causes an **increase in blood pressure.** Many studies show an association between active smoking and high blood pressure. A prospective study showed that the risk of high blood pressure in smokers (men) with more than 20 cigarettes per day is significantly higher (Dochi *et al.*, 2009). Another study in women similarly concluded that the risk of high blood pressure was increased in smokers who smoked 15 or more cigarettes per day (Bowman *et al.*, 2007).

Several studies have shown that hypertension is linked to risk factors:

Table III Some work on hypertension and its risk factors.

Author	Target population	Sample	Website	Results
(Sellam & Bour, 2016)	Moroccan women	624 women of childbearing age (aged 20-49), not pregnant, with no known medical condition	the prefecture of Oujda-Angad (Morocco)	Among the VRDFs recorded by this study: 30.6% obesity (BMI), 79.1% abdominal obesity (high waist circumference), 35% high blood pressure, 29% dyslipidaemia (22.9% hypercholesterolaemia, 18.6% hypertriglyceridaemia), 7.5% fasting hyperglycaemia, 6.2% type 2 diabetes, 35% metabolic syndrome -More than 33% of these women have one RDF, and more than 50% of women aged $\geq$ 40 years have more than three RDFs
(El Boukhrissi et al., 2017)	Military wives in the Meknes region, Morocco.	Sample of 800 women.	Moulay Ismail Military Hospital in Meknes (Morocco).	-The median age of the study population was 38 $\pm$ 5 years, the median waist circumference was 101.0 $\pm$ 8.53 cm, and the median BMI was 28.39 $\pm$ 3.11 kg/m2. -About 98% of the patients were abdominally obese. -The incidence of high blood pressure (BP) was 32%, while 27% of the participants had hyperglycaemia, and 18% had dyslipidaemia. -The frequency of VCDF increases with age, parity, low income and education. -The result obtained in this study suggests a considerable increase in cardiovascular diseases in the coming years.
(Hunt et al., 1991)		Sample of 482 normotensive adults.	The Cardiovascular Genetics Clinic at the University of Utah.	risk factors of age, body fat and height, plasma uric acid, phosphate and a family history of hypertension prospectively increase the risk of hypertension.

| (Perrine et al., 2019) | French population. | Sample of 2,169 adults aged 18-74 years. | Metropolitan France (excluding Corsica). | In this study :
 -The incidence of hypertension was 30.6% [95% CI: 28.1-33.2].
 -The incidence of hypertension was higher in men than in women (36.5% vs 25.2%) and increased with age.
 -Only 1 in 2 people were aware of their hypertension.
 -And of those with hypertension, 47.3% [45.1-54.8] were being treated with an antihypertensive drug. |

II.2.5 Complications :

If left untreated, diabetes and hypertension can lead to serious complications that affect many parts of the body and increase the overall risk of premature death.

High blood pressure can eventually lead to serious cardiovascular, cerebrovascular or target organ (kidney, retina, etc.) complications.

The main complications to which hypertensive people are exposed are: stroke, ischaemic heart disease (angina pectoris, myocardial infarction), arteriopathy of the lower limbs, chronic renal failure, retinopathy, neurodegenerative disease (Alzheimer's and related diseases) (Chraibi *et al.* 2012).

For diabetes, the main complications are: heart attack, stroke, kidney failure, leg amputation, vision loss and nerve damage. Thus, during pregnancy, poorly controlled diabetes increases the risk of intrauterine mortality and other complications (WHO, 2016).

Diabetes is frequently associated with hypertension. In fact, 80% of diabetics are hypertensive. This association multiplies the risk of cardiovascular complications. The frequency of coronary artery disease, stroke, neuropathy or retinopathy is twice as high in hypertensive diabetics compared to diabetics alone (NGENDAKUMANA, 2014).

II.2.6 Summary:

It appears from the different international studies that diabetes and hypertension are mainly influenced by: age, hypercholesterolemia, severe and moderate overweight and obesity, unbalanced diet, lack of physical activity, sedentary lifestyle, gender, high waist to hip ratio (WHR), heredity, smoking. So in our work we will test the associations between diabetes and hypertension and both diseases with some risk factors in a group of women.

II.3 Research question:

- Is there a relationship between certain chronic diseases (diabetes and hypertension) and the following risk factors: obesity, high cholesterol and age?

III. Materials and methods :

This work was carried out on a pre-established database by Prof. Maamri. The protocol followed in this research followed the following steps:

III.1 Study site :

The province of Berkane is located in the extreme North-East of the Kingdom and the Oriental region. It is bordered to the north by the Mediterranean Sea, to the east by the Moroccan-Algerian border and the prefecture of Oujda-Angad, to the west by the province of Nador and to the south by the province of Taourirt (Haut-Commissariat au Plan, 2017).

Covering a total area of 1985 km2, the province of Berkane represents 2.2% of the total area of the region. It is made up of 16 communes, 10 of which are rural, grouped into two circles: the circle of Ahfir, made up of 4 rural communes, and the circle of Aklim, made up of 6 rural communes (Haut-Commissariat au Plan, 2017).

According to the results of the 2014 General Census of Population and Housing, the province has 289137 inhabitants, i.e. 12.5% of the total population of the region with a density of 145.7 inhabitants/km2 (Haut-Commissariat au Plan, 2017).

The data collection was done in a health centre in the city of Berkane (Centre of Madagh) in the eastern region.

III.2 Type of study :

This is an epidemiological, cross-sectional, descriptive and analytical study conducted among women aged 18 to 85 years. The results presented in this work are based on data collected from a questionnaire including socio-demographic, anthropometric and biological characteristics (Maamri, 2019).

III.3 Study population:

We included in this survey female subjects, living in rural areas and aged 18 years and older on the day of the survey. We did not include pregnant or breastfeeding women, patients on insulin or corticosteroids, subjects who did not give their consent to participate in the survey, and persons unable to answer the questions.

III.4 Parameters studied :

Data were collected on the day of recruitment of the patients through questioning, physical examination and biological tests. The questioning made it possible to determine age, history of diabetes and arterial hypertension (age and current treatment).

Each patient underwent a complete somatic examination, including blood pressure and anthropometric measurements (weight, height and waist circumference (WC)).

The blood pressure was measured with a blood pressure monitor (OMRON) in the form of an inflatable cuff to be used on the arm, in a sitting or lying position. Hypertension is defined as having a systolic blood pressure greater than or equal to 140 mmHg and/or a diastolic blood pressure greater than or equal to 90 mmHg(WHO 2013a).

Overweight and obesity have been determined by calculating the Body Mass Index, which is expressed in Kg/m2 and is calculated according to the following formula

Weight (Kg)/ [Height (m) x Height (m)]

The WHO classification was used to identify the weight status of the patients (less than 18.5: Underweight (thin), 18.5 to 24.9: Normal weight, 25 to 29.9: Overweight, 30 to 34.5: Moderate obesity, 35 to 39.9: Severe obesity, more than 40: Morbid or massive obesity) (WHO, 2013). Weight was obtained using a mechanical scale in indoor clothing without shoes, and height was measured using a height gauge.

The waist circumference, also known as the abdominal circumference (or waist circumference), expressed in cm, measured halfway between the lower limit of the rib cage and the iliac crest, and the threshold at which the risk is increased varies according to the sex of the individual.

An individual with a waist circumference greater than or equal to 80cm was considered obese (WHO, 2013).

The biological assessment carried out for each patient included fasting blood glucose (FBG) or postprandial blood glucose (PPG), glycated haemoglobin (HbA1c), and lipid assessment (total cholesterol (TC), HDL cholesterol (HDL) and triglycerides (TG)).

Glycemic control was carried out by two twin blood tests of blood glucose levels:

- Glycated haemoglobin (HbA1C) which determines the concentration of glucose in the blood, the glycaemia, over three months. Any diabetic with an HbA1c $\geq$ 6.5% was considered to have unbalanced blood glucose (Nathan *et al.*, 2009).

Glycated haemoglobin was measured by an analyser (bioHermes) which allows the determination of glycated haemoglobin from a drop of blood by means of reagent cassettes.

- Fasting blood glucose, the level of glucose in the blood. It is measured in grams of glucose per litre of blood. If the blood sugar level is too high, it is called hyperglycaemia. If it is too low, it is called hypoglycaemia.

Fasting blood glucose was measured with a blood glucose meter (Caresens dual) by analysing a drop of blood, taken from the fingertip, using a self-prick pen. The blood sugar can be measured on an empty stomach or 1 to 2 hours after a meal. This is called "postprandial blood glucose". Any individual with a FPG$\geq$1.26g/l or GPP$\geq$2g/l is considered diabetic (Nathan *et al.*, 2009).

And for the lipid profile, cholesterol levels were measured by a cholesterol analyzer which allows the evaluation of LDL, HDL and total cholesterol levels, as well as triglycerides by a blood test (performed on an empty stomach). Cholesterol has been considered "normal" when it is below 2g/L (French Federation of Cardiology, 2020).

III.5 Statistical analysis :

The number of 150 women was randomly selected. The data were analysed using XLSTAT software.

In the descriptive study, for the univariate description we calculated absolute frequencies and relative frequencies (percentages) of different modalities for the qualitative variables. We calculated means and standard deviations for the quantitative variables. And for the bivariate description we described the association between the categorical variables by using a contingency table.

In the exploratory study on a large number of variables we used MCA (multiple correspondence analysis) to identify possible relationships between the different categorical variables.

In the analytical study, comparisons of 2 means on independent series were made by means of the ANOVA test. And the links between 2 qualitative variables were carried out by the Chi2 test on contingency table.

In all statistical tests, the significance level was set at 0.05.

III.6 Ethical considerations :

The protocol of the study was approved by the Ethics Committee for Biomedical Research in Oujda. All patients gave their oral consent after being explained the purpose of the work. Participation was voluntary and confidentiality was guaranteed, and in case of refusal to participate, this would not affect the person in any way. Participants were informed of their right to withdraw their consent or end their participation at any time. Participants who preferred not to answer certain questions were free to ignore them.

IV.   Results :

IV.1 Univariate analysis:

IV.1.1   Demographics :

Sex :

A total of 150 female subjects were included in this study, i.e. 100% of the sample

Age :

The age of the women surveyed ranged from 18 to 85 years, with an average of 50.84 years (standard deviation = 11.26 years) and a median of 50 years. The distribution of our sample by age group shows that the group studied is more represented by the 34-66 age group.

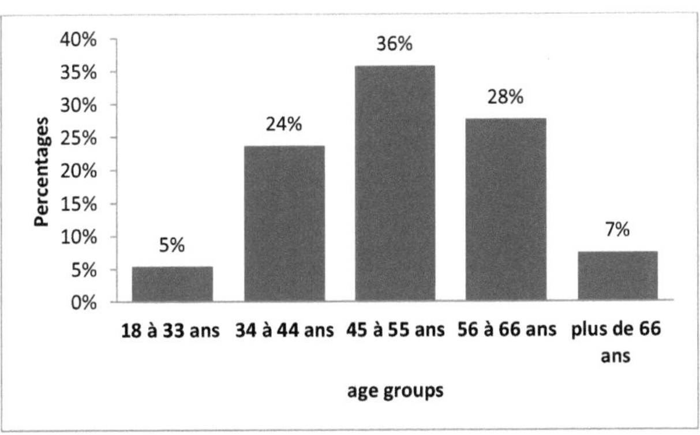

Figure 3Distribution of age groups in our overall sample .

IV.1.2   Anthropometric measurements :

Weight :

The mean weight was 74.1 kg (±13.2 kg) with a maximum weight of 110kg, a minimum weight of 46kg and a median of 75kg. The weight range >70kg was the most represented (62%).

Size :

The mean height of the overall sample was 1.57m (±0.09). The extremes were 1.05m for the minimum height and 1.72m for the maximum height and the median was 1.58m. The height ranges "1.50-1.59m" and "1.60-1.70m" were respectively the most represented at 55% and 37%.

Body Mass Index (BMI):

The body mass index ranged from 17.16kg.m-2 to 71.66kg.m-2 with a mean of 30.36 (±7.3) and a median of 29.75kg.m-2. In terms of frequencies, the results show that 30 individuals or 19% of the women studied were normo-weight, 46 (31%) were overweight and 74 (49%) were obese. The proportion of women with a BMI of less than 18.5 kg/m2 (underweight) was very low, at 1% (n=1). Among the obese women, we counted 46 women (30%) as moderately obese and 28 women (19%) as severely or morbidly obese.

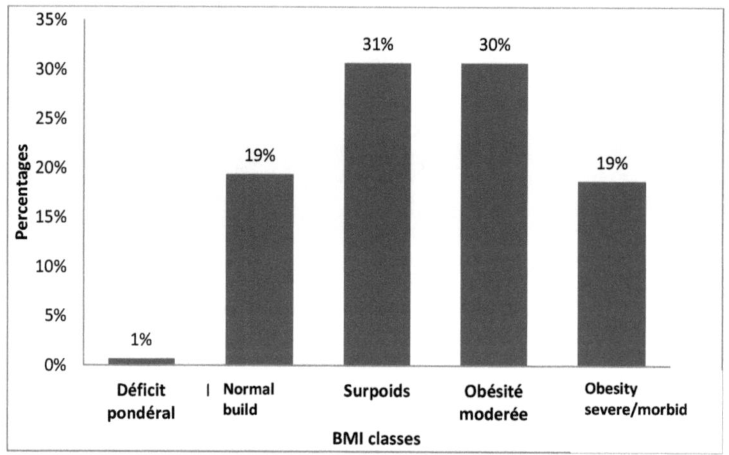

Figure 4 Distribution of the overall workforce by BMI .

The waist circumference of all the individuals collected ranged from 57cm to 184cm with a mean of 99.44cm (±14.22) and a median of 100cm. Of the subjects in the study, 139 individuals or 93% were obese according to their waist circumference.

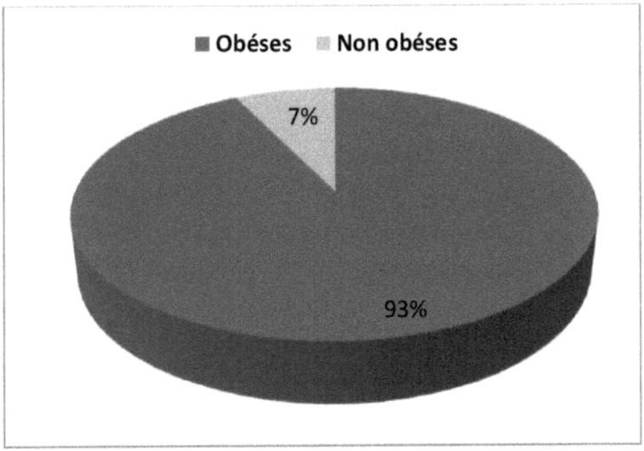

Figure 5 Distribution of the study sample according to abdominal obesity .

IV.1.3 Bioclinical measures :

Blood glucose :

Fasting blood glucose levels ranged from 4.64 to 0.52g/l and postprandial blood glucose levels from 1.84 to 1.12g/l. The results show that 38 individuals or 25% of the women studied were diabetic, and 112 or 75% non-diabetic. With 8 women or 21% of the diabetics being new cases.

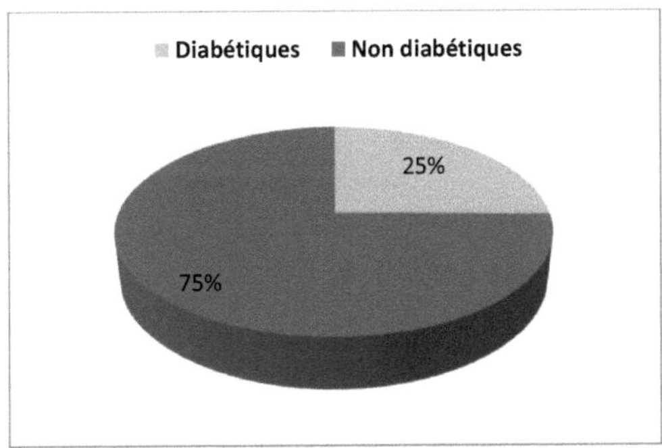

Figure 6 Distribution of participants according to blood glucose level.

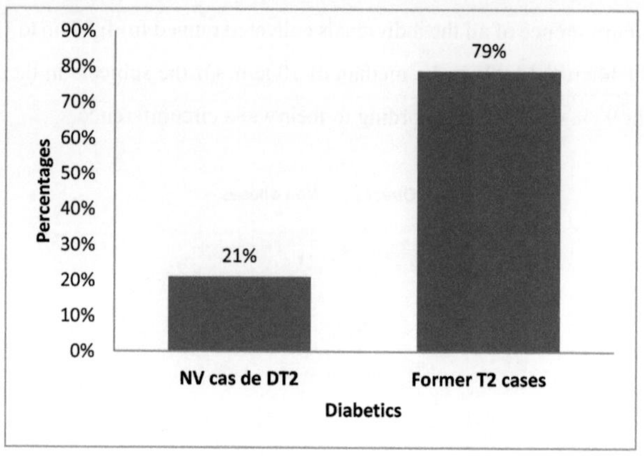

Figure 7Distribution of diabetics according to old and new cases.

Diabetes management :

We find that only 24% of diabetics show HbA1c values below 6.5% (balanced diabetes), while 76% show values above 6.5% (poor diabetes control).

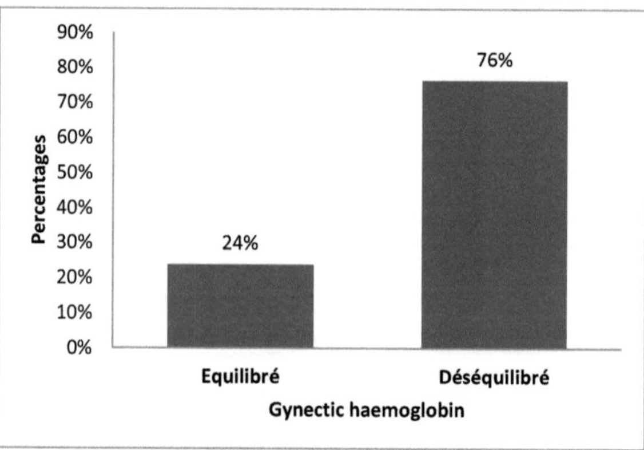

Figure 8 Distribution of diabetics according to glycated haemoglobin.

Concerning the treatment of diabetes, it was observed that only 45% of diabetics are under treatment.

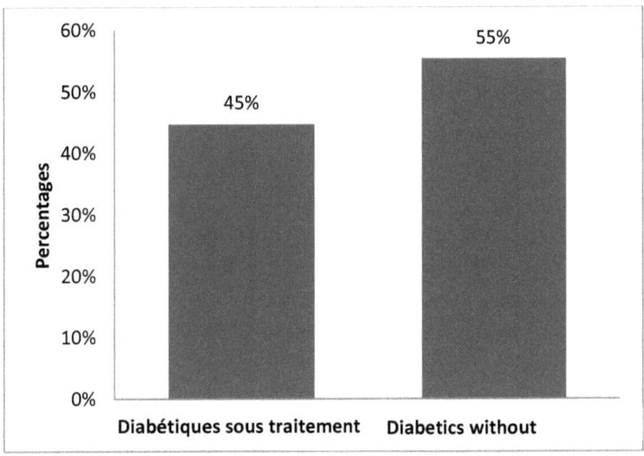

Figure 9 Distribution of diabetics according to diabetes treatment .

High blood pressure :

Systolic blood pressure ranged from 19mm Hg and 8mm Hg with a mean of 13.61mm Hg (±1.99) and a median of 13mm Hg. Diastolic blood pressure ranged from 11mm Hg and 6mm Hg with a mean of 8.09mm Hg (±1.09) and a median of 8mm Hg.

From a frequency perspective, the results show that 81 individuals or 54% of the women studied are hypertensive, and 69 (46%) are non-hypertensive.

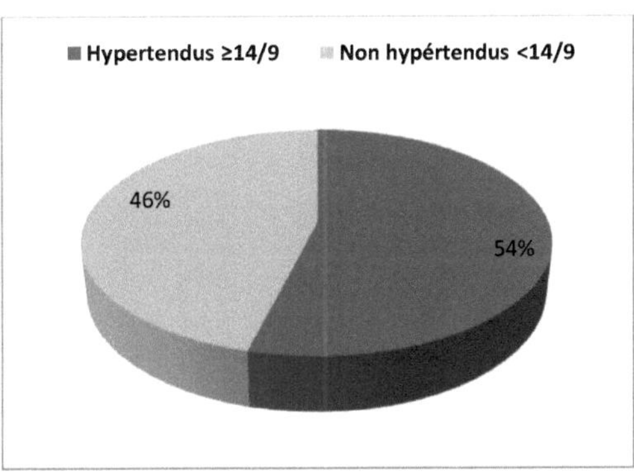

Figure 10 Distribution of participants according to high blood pressure.

Management of hypertension :

Regarding the management of hypertension, we find that among hypertensives, 61% are not undergoing treatment, while only 39% are undergoing treatment for hypertension.

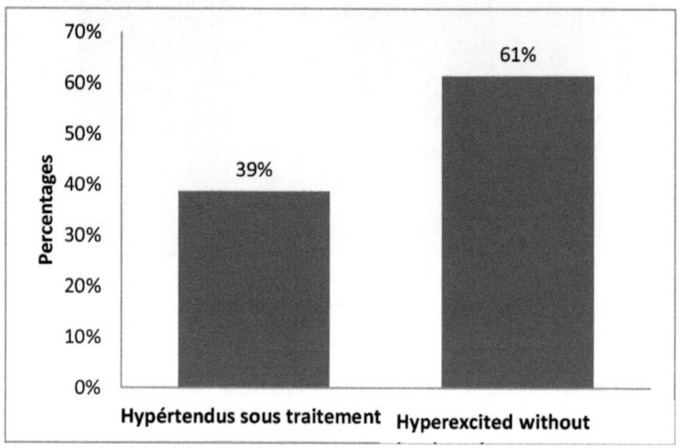

Figure 11 Distribution of hypertensive patients according to the treatment of hypertension .

The results show that 16% of the hypertensive women are new cases, 26% are former treated cases, and 58% are former untreated cases.

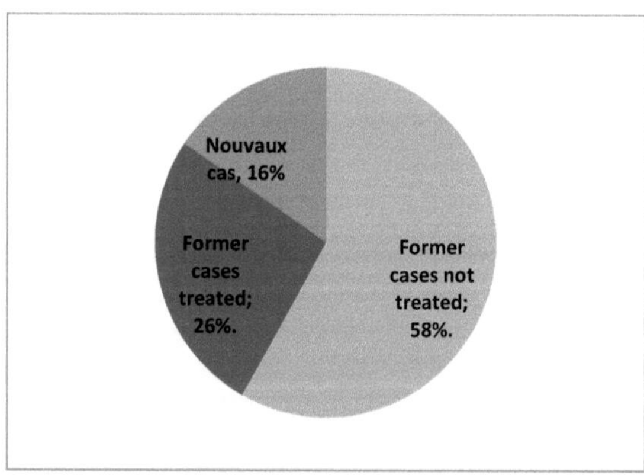

Figure 12 Distribution of participants according to the length of time they have had ATH.

Cholesterol levels ranged from 0.99 to 3.50g/l. The results show that 60 individuals or 40% of the women studied have high total cholesterol (>2g/l), while 90 individuals or 60% are normal.

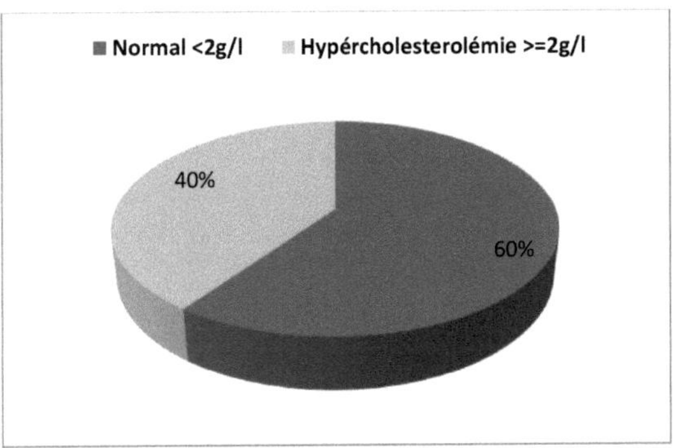

Figure 13Distribution of the overall workforce by cholesterol level.

IV.2 Multivariate analysis :

IV.2.1   MCA (multiple correspondence analysis) :

Table IV Cronbach's alpha reliability coefficient

		Variance Accounted For	
Dimension	Cronbach's Alpha	Total (Eigenvalue)	Inertia
1	,776	3,320	,332
2	,759	3,159	,316
Total		6,479	,648
Mean	,768[a]	3,239	,324

Model Summary

a. Mean Cronbach's Alpha is based on the mean Eigenvalue.

The Cronbach's alpha reliability coefficient is 0.76, which suggests that the items have a relatively high internal consistency.

Table V Eigenvalues and percentages of inertia :

	F1	F2	F3
Eigenvalue	0,3198	0,2320	0,2033
Inertia (%)	23,9823	17,3976	15,2449
Cumulative	23,9823	41,3800	56,6249
Adjusted inertia	0,0338	0,0061	0,0019
Adjusted inertia (%)	51,1381	9,3038	2,9224
Cumulative	51,1381	60,4418	63,3642

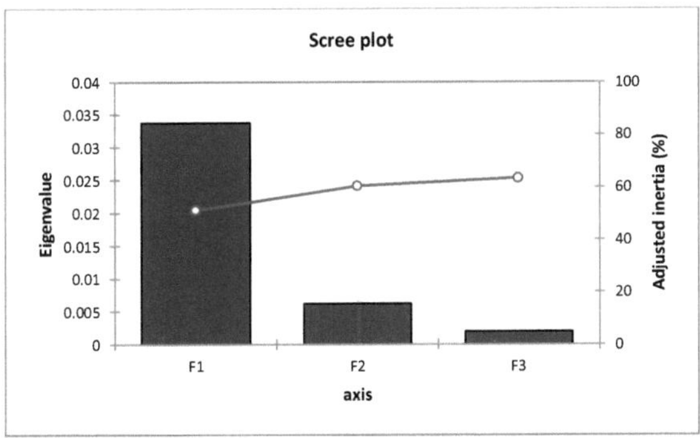

In the multiple correspondence analysis, axes F1 and F2 were chosen because they provide the most information, i.e. a percentage of inertia of 60.44%.

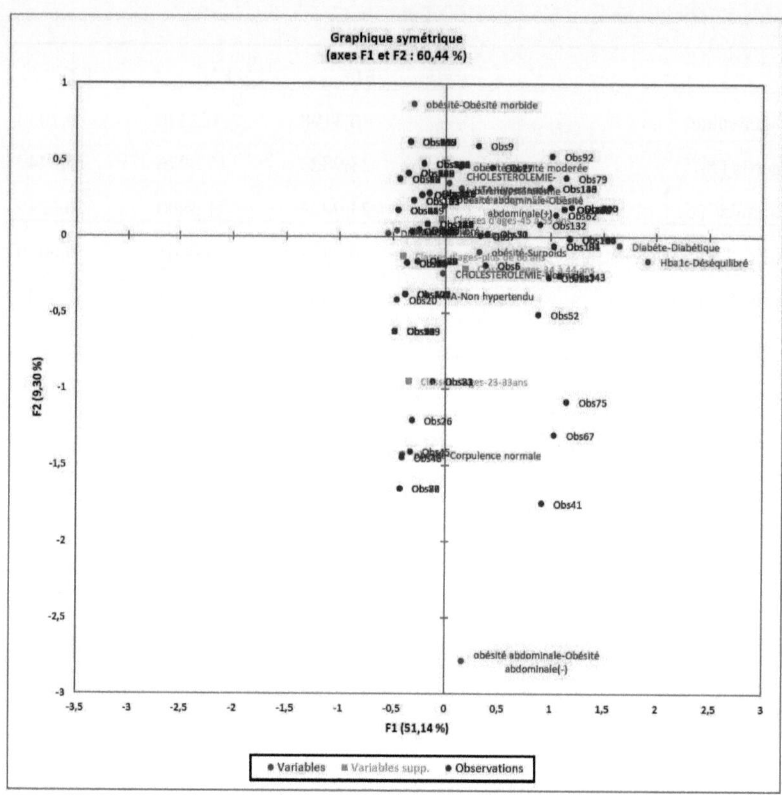

Graph I Symmetrical graph of observations-variables.

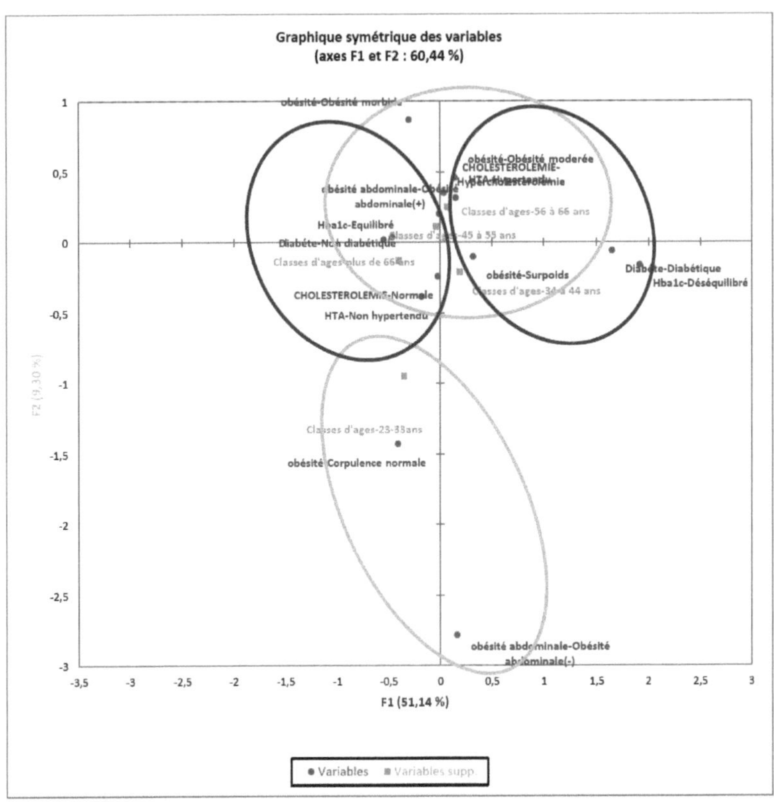

Graph IISymmetric graph of variables.

The results of the MCA show that :

The **F1** axis separates the group of diabetic women who have unbalanced Hba1c, hypercholesterolemia, and who are hypertensive. And the group of non-diabetic women, with normal cholesterol and balanced Hba1c and normal blood pressure. So the F1 axis is a diabetes-HTA axis.

The F2 axis separates two groups, one group of women who are 45 years and older, overweight or obese and have abdominal obesity. The other group is made up of women aged between 23 and 33 who are of normal build and do not have abdominal obesity. So the F2 axis is an obesity axis.

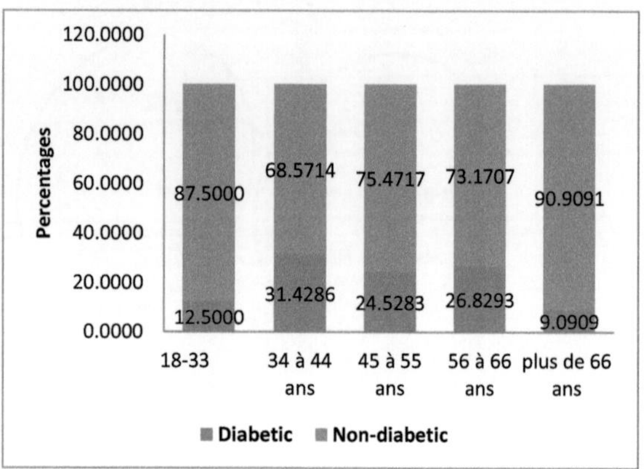

Figure 14Distribution of the overall sample by age group and diabetes.

The results show that diabetes mainly affects people aged 34 and over, but it should also be noted that even the younger age group is beginning to be affected by type 2 diabetes (12.50%). The most affected age group is 34 to 44 years (31.42%) and the least affected is the age group over 66 years with a percentage of 9.09%. With a significant difference in the distribution of age groups among diabetics P<0.0001, indicates the strong association between diabetes and age.

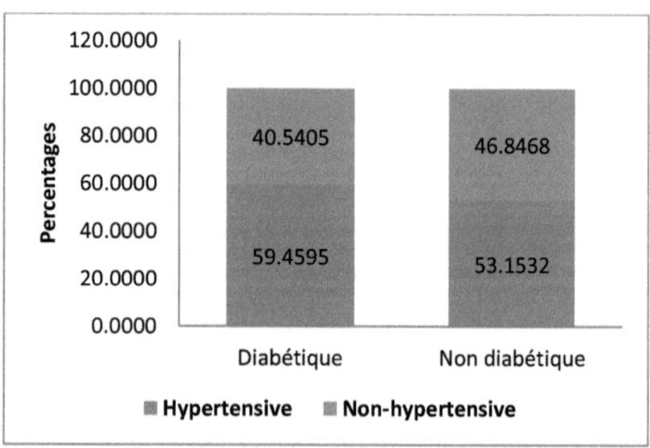

Figure 15Distribution of the overall sample according to hypertension and diabetes.

It was noted that hypertension was more prevalent in diabetics with a frequency of 59.45%, whereas in non-diabetics it represented only 53.15%. According to the results, a significant difference was found in the distribution of hypertensives among diabetics P<0.001, which indicates the strong association between these two pathologies.

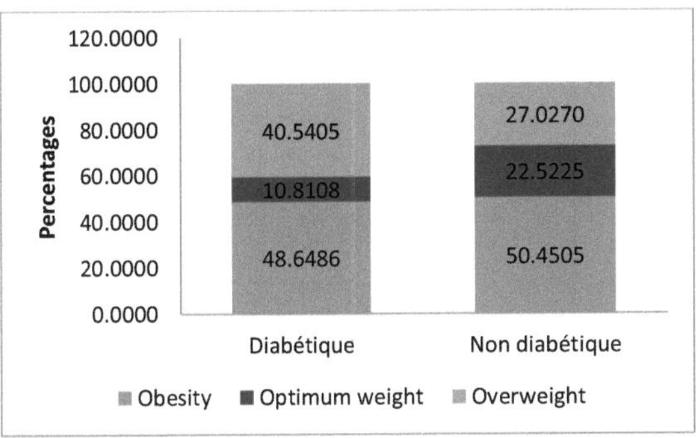

Figure 16Repair of the overall sample by obesity and diabetes.

From a frequency point of view, the results show that 48.64% of diabetics are obese, 40.54% are overweight and only 10.81% have a normal body shape. With a higher percentage of overweight among diabetics.

A highly significant difference was found in the distribution of BMI classes among diabetics P<0.00001 showing a significant association between obesity and diabetes.

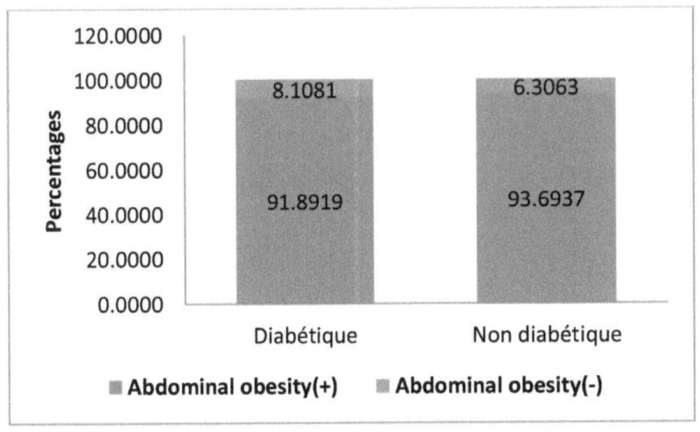

Figure 17Distribution of the overall sample by abdominal obesity and diabetes.

We find that 91.89% of diabetics are abdominally obese. With a significant difference in the distribution of abdominal obesity among diabetics P<0.001.

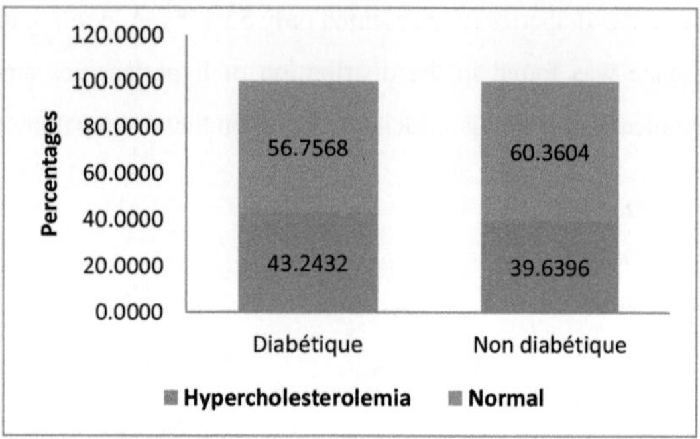

Figure 18Distribution of the overall sample by cholesterol and diabetes.

Hypercholesterolaemia was more present in diabetics with a frequency of 43.24% (39.63% in non-diabetics). A significant difference was found in the distribution of hypercholesterolaemia among diabetics P<0.001, indicating the association between diabetes and hypercholesterolaemia.

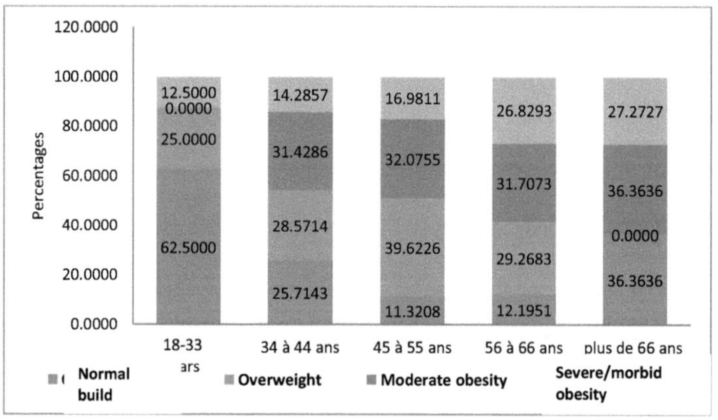

Figure 19Distribution of the overall sample by BMI classes and age groups .

The results show that obesity increases with age, and mainly affects those aged 56 and over. With a highly significant association between obesity and age P<0.0001.

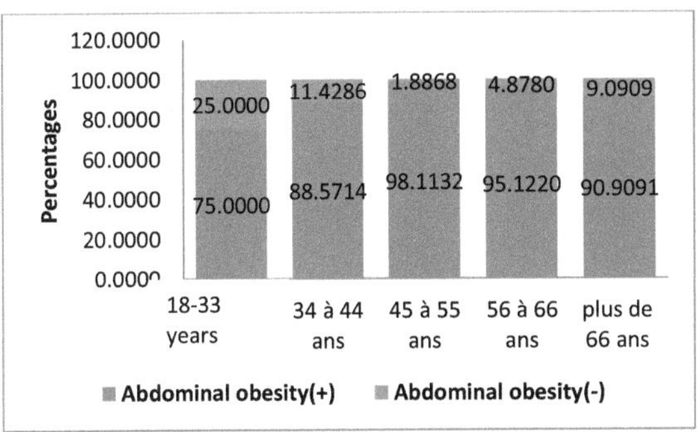

Figure 20Distribution of participants according to abdominal obesity and age groups .

Abdominal obesity was found in all age groups with very high percentages. The most affected age group was 45-55 years (98.11%), and the least affected was 18-33 years.The results show significant differences in the distribution of age groups within the obese according to waist circumference with a P<0.01 indicating a strong association between age and abdominal obesity.

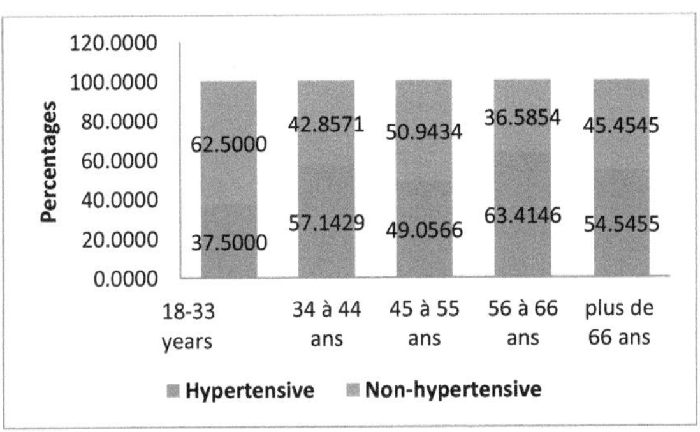

Figure 21Distribution of participants according to ATH and age groups .

Our results show that hypertension affects all age groups, mainly adults. The most affected age group is 56-66 years (63.41%) and the least affected is 18-33 years with a percentage of 37.50%. With a significant difference in the distribution of age groups within the hypertensive population P<0.001. This indicates a highly significant association between hypertension and age.

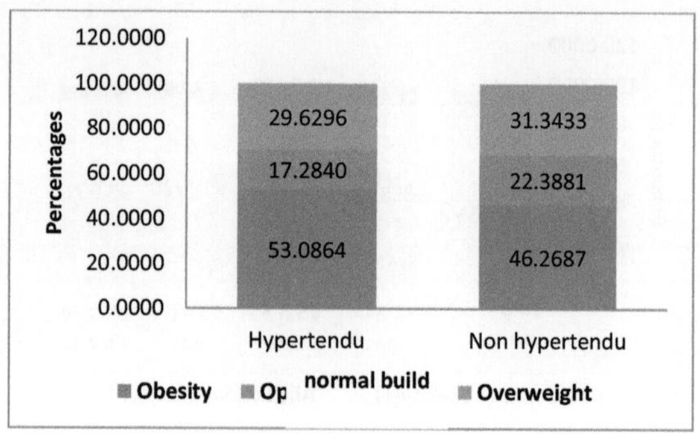

Figure 22Distribution of the study sample according to obesity and high blood pressure.

Among the hypertensive women, 53.08% were obese, 29.62% were overweight and only 17.28% were of normal build. A significant difference was detected in the distribution of BMI classes among the hypertensives P<0.001 which shows the significant association between obesity and hypertension.

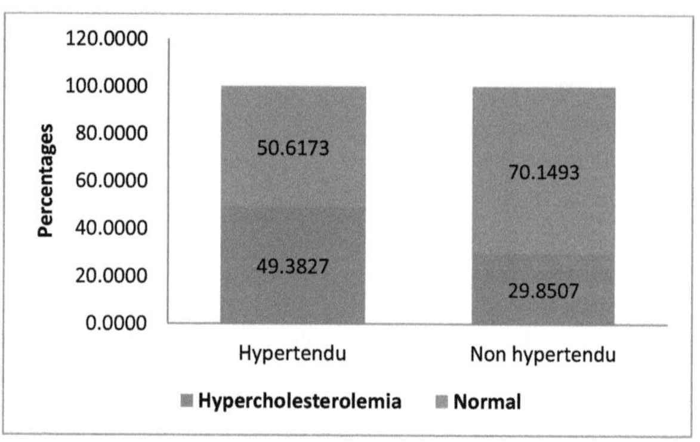

Figure 23Repair of participants according to cholesterol and 'HTA.

We observed that hypercholesterolemia was more present in hypertensives with a frequency of 49.38% (29.85% in non hypertensives).

Our results show a significant difference in the distribution of hypercholesterolaemia between hypertensives and non-hypertensives P=0.0160. In addition a significant difference was found in the distribution of hypercholesterolaemia within hypertensives P<0.0001.

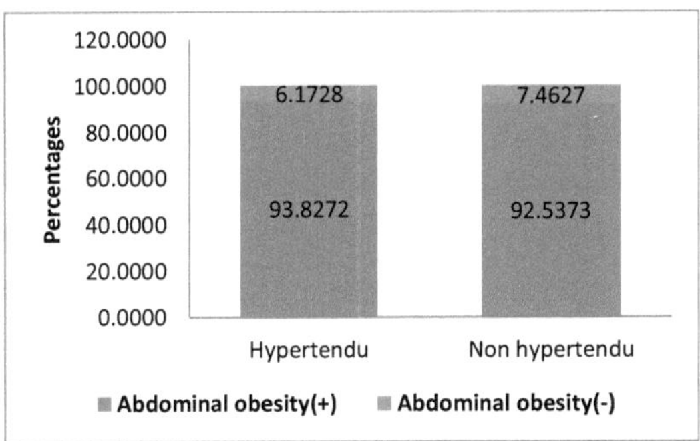

Figure 24Distribution of the overall sample by abdominal obesity and high blood pressure.

The incidence of abdominal obesity was higher in hypertensives 93.82. With a significant difference in the distribution of abdominal obesity within hypertensives P<0.01, showing that abdominal obesity has an effect on hypertension.

IV.2.3 Analysis of the association between the quantitative variables :

Concerning the comparison of the means of the quantitative variables. The results show no significant difference in the distribution of means within the two groups for all quantitative variables P>0.05, except for PAS (P=0.03).

V. Discussion:

In our study of a population of 150 women, 25% were found to be diabetic, well above the estimated national level of 10.6% (Belhadj et al., 2019). (Belhadj *et al.*, 2019). in 2017, it is estimated at 9.8% in Tunisia for the population aged 20 to 79 years. In 2018 it reached 14.4% in Algeria (Belhadj *et al.*, 2019). It was also noted that hypertension was detected in 54% of the study population, which is also much higher than that recorded in the study by Perrine *et* al. (Perrine *et al.*, 2019) and that recorded by the national survey on NCD risk factors (29.3%) in 2017 (Maamri & Ben El Mostafa, 2020).

The aim was to study the effect of risk factors, including obesity, on these two diseases. This was done on the basis of a questionnaire that included sociodemographic, anthropometric, and biological characteristics. It should be noted that our results may be at variance with previous work, which can be explained by differences in the samples and the working methods used.

As risk factors, obesity in all its forms was very present at relatively high rates in the overall sample: according to BMI the percentage of obese or overweight individuals was 80%, according to waist circumference this percentage was 93%. The frequency of obesity in our study (49%) is much higher than that recorded at the national level 20% (29% in women) (Maamri & Ben El Mostafa, 2020). This can be explained by the prestige associated with overweight and obesity, which symbolize social success, a sign of good health and prosperity, in the mentality of many people. these results are higher compared to other studies conducted in Morocco, such as that of Laayoune with an obesity frequency of (49%) (Rguibi & Belahsen, 2004)and that of Smara (43%) (Rahim & Baali, 2011).

In the comparison of the distribution of obesity among diabetics, 48.64% of diabetics were obese, 40.54% were overweight and only 10.81% had a normal body shape. According to the results, obesity in all its forms, either defined by BMI or waist circumference, showed significant differences (P<0.00001 for obesity; P<0.001 for abdominal obesity). A study in Bahrain shows this strong association between obesity and type 2 diabetes (Musaiger & Al-Mannai, 2002).

In the comparison of the distribution of obesity among hypertensive women, 53.08% of hypertensive women were obese, 29.62% were overweight and according to waist circumference this percentage was 93.82%. The results showed significant differences in the distribution of obesity and abdominal obesity among hypertensive women with P<0.001; P<0.01 respectively, which is in line with other works (Sellam & Bour, 2016;Bruckert, 2008;Ginsberg & Maccallum, 2009).

For cholesterol, the results showed that 40% of women had hypercholesterolemia, this result is higher than that of a study conducted in Oujda (22.9%) (Sellam & Bour, 2016). The distribution of our sample according to diabetes and hypercholesterolemia showed that 43.24% of diabetics had hypercholesterolemia, with a significant difference in the distribution of hypercholesterolemia within diabetics P<0.001. Several studies have shown this association between diabetes and hypercholesterolaemia (Benharrats & Bencharif, 2019;Mengesha, 2007).

Secondly, hypercholesterolaemia was present in 49.38% of hypertensive women. A significant difference in the distribution of hypercholesterolaemia was found between hypertensives and non-hypertensives P=0.0160. In addition, a significant difference was found in the distribution of hypercholesterolaemia within hypertensives P<0.0001. Several studies have shown this positive association between hypercholesterolaemia and increased hypertension (Cissé et al., 2016).

Furthermore, the distribution of our sample by age group revealed an overrepresentation of the 34-44/ 45-55/ 56-66 age group with a percentage of 23% and 35% and 27% respectively. Our results showed that obesity increases significantly with age P<0.0001. This has been demonstrated by other studies (Janghorbani et al., 2007;Zhang et al., 2008). Weight gain in older people can be explained by decreased physical activity (Gibson & Ferguson 1999)and by the decrease in metabolism that accompanies ageing (BM, 2002).

It was also noted that type 2 diabetes increases significantly with age P<0.0001 which is in line with several studies (Pan et al., 1997;Benharrats & Bencharif 2019;Musaiger & Al-Mannai 2002). But in our case it starts to manifest itself at an early age, this is due to several causes we can mention, the sedentary lifestyle (George, Rosenkranz, and Kolt 2013Rockette et al., 2015). A diet rich in fat, and less rich in slow sugar (Imamura et al.,

2009).

Analysis of the results showed that hypertension was more frequently encountered in older subjects than in younger ones, these results are statistically significant P<0.001, and are in agreement with other previous work (Hunt *et al.*, 1991;Perrine *et al.*, 2019).

We also found that 59.45% of diabetics were hypertensive, with a predominance of diabetics over non-diabetics. A comparison of the distribution of hypertension among diabetics showed a significant difference, P<0.001. All the series we consulted report this predominance of hypertension in diabetics, as is the case of Safi *et* al (2007). Diabetes is also recognized as a risk factor for the development of hypertension. According to a 2012 study, approximately 80% of T2DM patients will eventually develop hypertension (Scheen *et al.*, 2012). In fact, high blood pressure (BP) is one of the most common comorbidities. The coexistence of diabetes and hypertension increases the risk of cardiovascular disease, which is the major cause of death in diabetics (Normand, 2003).

As for the therapeutic management of diabetes and hypertension, only 45% of diabetics and 39% of hypertensives were on treatment, which is relatively low. The ENTRED study showed a frequency of treatment with oral antidiabetics of 87% in individuals under 65 years of age (Névanen *et al.*, 2001). This high frequency of non-adherence to treatment can be explained either by negligence or lack of knowledge, of which 16% of hypertensives and 21% of diabetics are new cases, which has very serious repercussions because diabetes and hypertension can lead to other pathologies.

HbA1c measurement is a more relevant element for monitoring glycaemic control in diabetics than fasting blood glucose, which is only a snapshot. Only 24% of diabetics have a balanced hbA1c. This result shows that the majority of the patients studied have unbalanced diabetes. This can be explained by non-compliance with diet and hygiene prescriptions. A randomised study by the UKPDS clearly showed the link between increased HbA1c and an exponential increase in the risk of complications (Turner, 1998).

Conclusion

In the light of the results obtained we can conclude that :

The frequencies of diabetes and hypertension were very high in the population of women studied. As risk factors, obesity was found in 49%, overweight in 31% and abdominal obesity in 40% of the women studied.

Diabetes and hypertension were mainly related to age, obesity, abdominal obesity, and hypercholesterolemia. There was a statistically significant association between these two conditions. This study raises the need for increased prevention programmes against these diseases in our populations unable to cope with the complications that may arise, and opens up prospects for the prevention and reduction of the risk of diabetes and hypertension and blood glucose control.

It is therefore necessary to monitor oneself regularly throughout one's life, to maintain good eating and physical activity habits, and to take medication regularly and appropriately. At the price of this daily constraint, diabetes is very well controlled, most complications are prevented and life expectancy increases.

Reference :

Abdelhay, B. (2017) -The effects of the Mediterranean diet on chronic diseases: Cardiovascular diseases, oxidative stress, dyslipidemia, diabetes mellitus, blood pressure, cancer, neurodegenerative diseases and obesity. Nutrition Research Reviews (ISSN: 0954-4224, ESSN: 1475-2700). https://hal.archives-ouvertes.fr/hal-01629438.

André,G. (2004) -Diabetes type II. Elsevier. 504p, ISBN: 2842996151, 9782842996154.

Arbouche, Belhadj, Berrah, Brouri, Kaddache, Khalfa, Malek, Semrouni (2012) - L'essentiel en diabetologie : à l'usage des medecins generalistes (SANOFI ed.). 9th congress of the Maghreb Federation of Endocrinology- Diabetology.

Balkau, B. Lange, C. Fezeu, L. Tichet, J. Blandine, D. Czernichow, S. Fumeron, F. Froguel, P *et al.* (2008) -'Predicting diabetes: Clinical, biological, and genetic approaches'. Diabetes Care. 31(10), pp. 2056-2061. doi: 10.2337/dc08-0368.

Belhadj, M. Lhassani, H. Khochtali, I. (2019) -'Management of type 2 diabetes in the Maghreb: Current state'. Medecine des Maladies Metaboliques. Elsevier Masson SAS, 13, pp. eS4-eS7. doi: 10.1016/S1957-2557(19)30198-1.

Benharrats, S. S. Bencharif, M. A. (2019) -'Comorbidity schizophrenia and diabetes mellitus in Algeria - A study of risk factors'. Revue d'Epidemiologie et de Sante Publique. Elsevier Masson SAS, 67(3), pp. 189-197. doi: 10.1016/j.respe.2019.02.005.

Bessire, N. (2000) - Diabetic ketoacidosis and pregnancy. Thesis n° 10093, Faculty of Medicine, University of Geneva.

BM, P. (2002) -'An overview on the nutrition transition and its health implications: the Bellagio meeting'. Public Health Nutrition. Cambridge University Press (CUP), 5(1a), pp. 93-103. doi: 10.1079/phn2001280.

Bowman, T. S. Gaziano, J. M. Buring, J. E. Sesso, H. D. (2007) - 'A Prospective Study of Cigarette Smoking and Risk of Incident Hypertension in Women'. Journal of the American College of Cardiology. J Am Coll Cardiol, 50(21), pp. 2085-2092. doi:10.1016/j.jacc.2007.08.017.

Bruckert, É. (2008) -'L'obésité abdominale: une menace pour la santé', Presse Medicale. Elsevier Masson, 37(10), pp. 1407-1414. doi: 10.1016/j.lpm.2008.01.021.

CAMBOU, J. P. (2010) Fréquence de l'hypertension selon l'âge. réalités Cardiologiques.

Cissé, F. Agne, F. Diatta, A. Mbengue, A. S. Ndiaye, A. Samba, A. Thiam, S. Doupa, D. Sarr, G. Sall, N. D. Touré, M. (2016) -'Prevalence of dyslipemia in Aristide le Dantec biochemistry laboratory in Dakar Senegal'. The Pan African medical journal. African Field Epidemiology Network, 25, p. 67. doi: 10.11604/pamj.2016.25.67.7758.

Chraibi, N. Zaid, D. Habbal, R. Batalha, S. Achibet, A. (2012) -Recommendations of Good Medical Practice Adult Hypertension, Guide du Praticien. Ministry of Health. ISBN: 978 - 9954 - 0 - 8548 - 6.

Daousi, C. Casson, I. F. Gill, G. V. MacFarlane, I. A.Wilding, J. P.H. Pinkney, J. H. (2006) 'Prevalence of obesity in type 2 diabetes in secondary care: Association with cardiovascular risk factors'. Postgraduate Medical Journal. BMJ Publishing Group, 82(966), pp. 280-284. doi: 10.1136/pmj.2005.039032.

Dembele, M. Sidibe, A. T. Traore, H. A. Tchombou, H. Zounet, B. Traore, A.K. Diallo, D. Fongoro, S (2000) -'ASSOCIATION HTA-DIABETE SUCRE DANS LE SERVICE DE MEDECINE INTERNE DE L'HOPITAL DU POINT G-BAMAKO'. Médecine d'Afrique Noire, 47(6).

Direction des statistiques (2011) l'enquête nationale sur les niveaux de vie des ménages marocains en 1998/1999.

Diyane, K. El Ansari, N. El Mghari, G. Anzid, K. Cherkaoui, M. (2013) 'Characteristics of the association of type 2 diabetes and hypertension in subjects aged 65 years and above'. Pan African Medical Journal. African Field Epidemiology Network, 14. doi:10.11604/pamj.2013.14.100.1880.

Dochi, M. Sakata, K. Oishi, M. Tanaka, K. Kobayashi, E. Suwazono, Y. (2009) 'Smoking as an independent risk factor for hypertension: A 14-year longitudinal study in male

Japanese workers'. Tohoku Journal of Experimental Medicine. Tohoku J Exp Med, 217(1), pp. 37-43. doi: 10.1620/tjem.217.37.

El Boukhrissi, F. Bamou, Y. Ouleghzal, H. Safi, S. Balouch, L. (2017) -'Prevalence of risk factors for cardiovascular disease and metabolic syndrome among women in the region of Meknes, Morocco', Medicine of Metabolic Diseases. Elsevier Masson SAS, 11(2), pp. 188-194. doi: 10.1016/S1957-2557(17)30047-0.

Fafa, N. Meskine, D. Kedad, L. Fedala, S. Heddam, A.E.M. Tobal, Z. (2015) 'Determinants of obesity in an Algiers population', Annals of Endocrinology. Elsevier BV, 76(4), p. 562. doi: 10.1016/j.ando.2015.07.888.

French Federation of Cardiology. (2020) -Cholesterol. https://www.fedecardio.org/Je-m-informe/Reduire-le-risque-cardio-vasculaire/le-cholesterol.

French Federation of Cardiology. (2019a) - ACTING AGAINST CHOLESTEROL TO REDUCE CARDIO-VASCULAR RISKS.

French Federation of Cardiology. (2019b) -ARTERIAL HYPERTENSION FIRST CARDIO-VASCULAR RISK FACTOR.

Feinleib, M. Garrison, R. J. Fabsitz, R. Christian, J. C. Hrubec, Z. Borhani, N. O. Kannel, W. B. Rosenman, R. Schwartz, J. T. Wagner, J. O. (1977) 'The nhlbi twin study of cardiovascular disease risk factors: Methodology and summary of results', American Journal of Epidemiology. Oxford University Press, 106(4), pp. 284-295. doi:10.1093/oxfordjournals.aje.a112464.

Fletcher, B., Gulanick, M. Lamendola, C. (2002) 'Risk factors for type 2 diabetes mellitus'. Journal of Cardiovascular Nursing, 16(2), p. 486. doi: 10.1097/00005082-200201000-00003.

Futura-sciences (2018) Cholesterol levels: high cholesterol and consequences. www.futura-sciences.com.

George, E. S., Rosenkranz, R. R. Kolt, G. S. (2013) 'Chronic disease and sitting time in middle-aged Australian males: Findings from the 45 and Up Study'. International Journal of Behavioral Nutrition and Physical Activity. BioMed Central, 10(1), p. 20. doi: 10.1186/1479-5868-10-20.

Gibson, R. S. Ferguson, E. L. (1999) -An interactive 24-hour recall for assessing the adequacy of iron and zinc intakes in developing countries. Press.

Ginsberg, H. N. Maccallum, P. R. (2009) 'The obesity, metabolic syndrome, and type 2 diabetes mellitus pandemic: Part I. Increased cardiovascular disease risk and the importance of atherogenic dyslipidemia in persons with the metabolic syndrome and type 2 diabetes mellitus', Journal of the Cardiometabolic Syndrome. NIH Public Access, pp. 113-119. doi: 10.1111/j.1559-4572.2008.00044.x.

Girerd, X. Murino, M. (2007) 'FLAHS studies: a dashboard of the epidemiology of hypertension in France (Comité Français de Lutte contre l'Hypertension Artériel)'. FRANCE, 306, pp. 6-9. www.comitehta.org.

Hajar, R. (2016) -THE MANAGEMENT AND TREATMENT OF TYPE 2 DIABETES . FACULTY OF MEDICINE AND PHARMACY OF RABAT, THESIS N°: 43.

Haut-Commissariat au Plan (2017) -Monography of the province of Berkane.

Hu, F. B. Manson, J. E. Stampfer, M. J. Colditz, G. Liu, S. Solomon, C. G. Willett, W. C. (2001) 'Diet, lifestyle, and the risk of type 2 diabetes mellitus in women', New England Journal of Medicine, 345(11), pp. 790-797. doi: 10.1056/NEJMoa010492

Hunt, S. C. Stephenson, S. H. Hopkins, P. N. Williams, R. R. (1991) 'Predictors of an increased risk of future hypertension in Utah: A screening analysis', Hypertension. Lippincott Williams and Wilkins, 17(6 SUPPL. 2), pp. 969-976. doi: 10.1161/01.hyp.17.6.969.

Imamura, F. Lichtenstein, A. H. Dallal, G. E. Meigs, J. B. Jacques, P. F. (2009) 'Generalizability of dietary patterns associated with incidence of type 2 diabetes mellitus', American Journal of Clinical Nutrition, 90(4), pp. 1075-1083. doi: 10.3945/ajcn.2009.28009

Janghorbani, M. Amini, M. Willett, W. C. Gouya, M. M. Delavari, A. Alikhani, S. Mahdavi, A. (2007) 'First nationwide survey of prevalence of overweight, underweight, and abdominal obesity in Iranian adults', Obesity. Obesity (Silver Spring), 15(11), pp. 2797-2808. doi: 10.1038/oby.2007.332.

Kearney, P. M. Whelton, M. Reynolds, K. Muntner, P. Whelton, P. K. He, J. (2005) 'Global burden of hypertension: analysis of worldwide data', The Lancet. Elsevier BV, 365(9455), pp. 217-223. doi: 10.1016/s0140-6736(05)17741-1.

Lotfi, Z. Aboussaleh, Y. Sbaibi, R. Achouri, I. Benguedour, R. (2017) 'Overweight, obesity and glycemic control among diabetics at the provincial diabetes reference centre (CRD), Kenitra, Morocco', Pan African Medical Journal. African Field Epidemiology Network, 27. doi: 10.11604/pamj.2017.27.189.9535.

Maamri, A. Ben El Mostafa, S. (2020) 'The environmental health role in reducing non communicable diseases through a healthy lifestyle', in Disease Prevention and Health Promotion in Developing Countries. Springer International Publishing, pp. 39-59. doi: 10.1007/978-3-030-34702-4_4.

Mazouni, FZ. Iferghas, A, Berri H, Maaroufi, A. (2018) bulletin d'epidémiologie et de santé publique, Programme National de Prévention et de Contrôle du Diabète, minister de la santé.(50).

Mengesha, A. Y. (2007) 'Hypertension and related risk factors in type 2 diabetes mellitus (DM) patients in Gaborone City Council (GCC) clinics, Gaborone, Botswana.', African health sciences. Makerere University Medical School, 7(4), pp. 244-245. http://www.nhlbi.nih.gov/about/.

Ministry of Health. (2016) - Moroccan nutrition guide.

Ministry of Health. (2018) -REPORT OF THE NATIONAL SURVEY ON COMMON RISK FACTORS FOR NON-COMMUNICABLE DISEASES 2017-2018.

Ministry of Health (2000) World High Blood Pressure Day. https://www.sante.gov.ma/Pages/SanteNews.aspx?IDSnews=21.

Ministry of Health. (2011) -The National Nutrition Strategy 2011-2019.

Musaiger, A. O. Al-Mannai, M. A. (2002) 'Social and lifestyle factors associated with diabetes in the adult Bahraini population', Journal of Biosocial Science. Cambridge University Press, 34(2), pp. 277-281. doi: 10.1017/s0021932002002778.

Nathan, D. M. Balkau, B. Bonora, E. Borch-Johnsen, K. Buse, J. B. Colagiuri, S. Davidson, M. B. DeFronzo, R. Genuth, S. Holman, R. R. Ji, L. Kirkman, S. Knowler, W. C. Schatz, D. Shaw, J. Sobngwi, E. Steffes, M. Vaccaro, O. Wareham, N. Zinman, B. Kahn, R. (2009) 'International expert committee report on the role of the A1C assay in the diagnosis of diabetes', Diabetes Care. American Diabetes Association, pp. 1327-1334. doi: 10.2337/dc09-9033.

Nejjari, C. Arharbi, M. Chentir, M. T. Boujnah, R. Kemmou, O. Megdiche, H. Boulahrouf, F. Messoussi, K. Nazek, L. Bulatov, V. (2013) 'Epidemiological Trial of Hypertension in North Africa (ETHNA): An international multicentre study in Algeria, Morocco and Tunisia', Journal of Hypertension. Lippincott Williams and Wilkins, 31(1), pp. 49-62. doi:10.1097/HJH.0b013e32835a6611.

Névanen, S. Tambekou, J. Fosse, S. Simon, D.Weill, A. Varroud-Vial, M *et al.* (2001) Characteristics and health status of elderly diabetics and their medical management, Entred 2001 study. BEH 2005, pp. 51-52.

New, J. P. Mason, J. M. Freemantle, N. Teasdale, S. Wong, L. M. Bruce, N. J. Burns, J. A. Gibson, J. M. (2003) 'Specialist nurse-led intervention to treat and control hypertension and hyperlipidemia in diabetes (SPLINT): A randomized controlled trial', Diabetes Care. Diabetes Care, 26(8), pp. 2250-2255. doi: 10.2337/diacare.26.8.2250.

Ngendakumana, E. (2014) -Evaluation of hypertension control by ABPM in hypertensive diabetic patients, THESIS.

Normand Racine (2003) 'L'hypertension artérielle chez le patient diabétiques', le clinicien.
http://www.stacommunications.com/journals/pdfs/clinicien/pdfclinicienfeb03/DrRacine hpertension.pdf.

WHO. (2002) 'World Health Report', World Health Organization.

WHO. (2013a) -Hypertension: a public health problem.

WHO. (2013b) - World Health Day 2013: control your blood pressure, control your life.

WHO. (2020) - Key benchmarks on obesity and overweight.

World Health Organization. (2013) -Global Overview of Hypertension.

World Health Organization. (2016) 'GLOBAL DIABETES REPORT'.

World Health Organization. (2003) -Obesitis: prevention and management of the global epidemic: report of a WHO consultation. World Health Organization.

World Health Organization. (2013) -Global action plan for the control of non-communicable diseases (2013-2020). Geneva. http://www.who.int/nmh/events/2012/action_plan_20120726_fr.pdf.

World Health Organization. (2016) -WORLD REPORT ON DIABETES. www.who.int.

Pan, X. Li, G. Hu, Y. Wang, J. Yang, W. An, Z. Hu, Z. Lin, J. Xiao, J. Cao, H. Liu, P. Jiang, X. Jiang, Y. Wang, J. Zheng, H. Zhang, H. Bennett, P. H. Howard, B. V. (1997) 'Effects of diet and exercise in preventing NIDDM in people with impaired glucose tolerance: The Da Qing IGT and diabetes study', Diabetes Care. American Diabetes Association Inc, 20(4), pp. 537-544. doi: 10.2337/diacare.20.4.537.

Pan, X., Yang, W. Liu, J. (1997) 'Prevalence of diabetes and its risk factors in China 1994. National Diabetes Prevention and Control Cooperative Group', Zhonghua nei ke za zhi [Chinese journal of internal medicine]. Diabetes Care, 36(6), pp. 384-389. doi: 10.2337/diacare.20.11.1664.

Perrine, A.-L. Lecoffre, C. Blacher, J. Olié, V. (2019) 'Hypertension in France: prevalence, treatment and control in 2015 and evolutions since 2006 ', Revue de Biologie Médicale.

Philippe, J. (2014) Study of monogenic forms of type 2 diabetes and obesity by next generation sequencing. Université Lille 2 Droit et Santé, Faculté de Médecine de Lille.

https://tel.archives-ouvertes.fr/tel-01198926.

Punthakee, Z., Goldenberg, R. Katz, P. (2018) 'Definition, Classification and Diagnosis of Diabetes, Prediabetes and Metabolic Syndrome', Canadian Journal of Diabetes. Elsevier B.V., 42, pp. S10-S15. doi: 10.1016/j.jcjd.2017.10.003.

Rahim, S. Baali, A. (2011) 'Étude de l'obésité et quelques facteurs associes chez un groupe de femmes marocaines résidentes de la ville de Smara (sud du Maroc)', Antropo, 24, pp. 43-53. www.didac.ehu.es/antropo.

Rguibi, M. Belahsen, R. (2004) 'Metabolic syndrome among Moroccan Sahraoui adult women', American Journal of Human Biology. Am J Hum Biol, 16(5), pp. 598-601. doi: 10.1002/ajhb.20065.

Rockette-Wagner, B. Edelstein, S. Venditti, E. M. Reddy, D. Bray, G. A. Carrion-Petersen, M. Dabelea, D. Delahanty, L. M. Florez, H. Franks, P. W. Montez, M. G. Rubin, R. Kriska, A. M. (2015) 'The impact of lifestyle intervention on sedentary time in individuals at high risk of diabetes', Diabetologia. Springer Verlag, 58(6), pp. 1198-1202. doi: 10.1007/s00125-015-3565-0.

Safi, S. Balouch, L. Hassikou, H. Sbiti, M. Ait Lhaj, H. Bamou, Y. Hadri, L. (2007) 'Magnesium status in a Moroccan population of type 2 diabetic patients', Cahiers de Nutrition et de Dietetique. Elsevier Masson SAS, 42(1), pp. 37-41. doi: 10.1016/s0007-9960(07)88698-6.

Scheen, A. J., Philips, J.-C. Krzesinski, J.-M. (2012) 'Hypertension and diabetes: about a common but complex association', Rev Med Liege, 67(3), pp. 133-138.

Sellam, E. B. Bour, A. (2016a) 'Obesity and hypertension in women of childbearing age in Morocco Obesity and hypertension in women of childbearing age in Morocco', Antropo, 36, pp. 57-66.www.didac.ehu.es/antropo.

Sellam, E. B. Bour, A. (2016b) 'Prevalence of risk factors for cardiovascular disease in women in Oujda (Morocco)', Medicine of Metabolic Diseases. Elsevier Masson SAS, 10(1), pp. 63-69. doi: 10.1016/S1957-2557(16)30020-7.

Shaw, J. E., Sicree, R. A. Zimmet, P. Z. (2010) 'Global estimates of the prevalence of diabetes for 2010 and 2030', Diabetes Research and Clinical Practice, pp. 4-14. doi: 10.1016/j.diabres.2009.10.007.

Simon, D. Eschwege, E. (2002) -'Epidemiological data on type 2 diabetes'. Bulletin Epidémiologique Hebdomadaire, 20, pp. 86-86.

Staessen, J. A. Wang, J. Bianchi, G. Birkenhäger, W. H. (2003) 'Essential hypertension', in Lancet. Elsevier Limited, 361(9369), pp. 1629-1641. ISSN: 01406736, doi: 10.1016/S0140-6736(03)13302-8.

Tenenbaum, M. Bonnefond, A. Froguel, P. Abderrahmani, A. (2018) 'Physiopathology of diabetes', Revue Francophone des Laboratoires,(502), pp. 26-32. doi: 10.1016/S1773-035X(18)30145-X.

Tuomilehto, J. Lindström, J. Eriksson, J. G. Valle, T. T. Hamäläinen, H. Ianne-Parikka, P. Keinänen-Kiukaanniemi, S. Laakso, M. Louheranta, A. Rastas, M. Salminen, V. Uusitupa, M. (2001) 'Prevention of type 2 diabetes mellitus by changes in lifestyle among subjects with impaired glucose tolerance', New England Journal of Medicine. N Engl J Med, 344(18), pp. 1343-1350. doi: 10.1056/NEJM200105033441801.

Turner, R. (1998) 'Effect of intensive blood-glucose control with metformin on complications in overweight patients with type 2 diabetes (UKPDS 34)', Lancet. Elsevier Limited, 352(9131), pp. 854-865. doi: 10.1016/S0140-6736(98)07037-8.

Vazquez, G. Duval, S. Jacobs, D. R. Silventoinen, K. (2007) 'Comparison of body mass index, waist circumference, and waist/hip ratio in predicting incident diabetes: A meta-analysis'. Epidemiologic Reviews. 29(1), pp. 115-128. doi: 10.1093/epirev/mxm008.

Villar, E. Zaoui, P. (2010) 'Diabetes and chronic kidney disease: Lessons from renal epidemiology', Nephrology and Therapeutics. Elsevier Masson SAS. 6(7), pp. 585-590. doi: 10.1016/j.nephro.2010.08.002.

WAGNER, A. ARVEILER, D. RUIDAVETS, J.B. COTTEL, D. BONGARD, V. DALLONGEVILLE, J. FERRIERES, J. AMOUYEL, P. HAAS, B. (2008) 'Etat des lieux sur l'hypertension artérielle en France en 2007 : l'étude Mona Lisa', Bulletin épidémiologique hebdomadaire, pp, 49-50, ISSN: 0245-7466.

WHO/FAO. (2003) -Diet, nutrition and the prevention of chronic diseases: Recommendations for preventing excess weight gains and obesity.

WHO EMRO. (2013) -Hypertension: a public health problem, World Health Day.

Yayehd, K. Damorou, F. Akakpo, R. Tchérou, T. N'Da, N. W. Pessinaba, S. Belle, L. Johnson, A. (2013) 'Prevalence of arterial hypertension and description of its risk factors in Lomé (Togo): Results of a screening conducted in the general population in May 2011', Annals of Cardiology and Angeiology, 62(1), pp. 43-50. doi:10.1016/j.ancard.2012.09.006.

Zhang, X. Sun, Z. Zhang, X. Zheng, L. Liu, S. Xu, C. Li, J. Zhao, F. Li, J. Hu, D. Sun, Y. (2008) 'Prevalence and associated factors of overweight and obesity in older rural Chinese', Internal Medicine Journal. Intern Med J, 38(7), pp. 580-586. doi: 10.1111/j.1445-5994.2007.01529.x.

Table VI Table of contributions.

	Weight	Weight (relative)	F1	F2	F3
Diabetic	37	0,0417	0,3540	0,0006	0,0002
Non-diabetic	111	0,1250	0,1180	0,0002	0,0001
Moderate obesity	45	0,0507	0,0032	0,0464	0,0781
Morbid obesity	29	0,0327	0,0095	0,1066	0,0665
Normal build	29	0,0327	0,0172	0,2871	0,0629
Overweight	45	0,0507	0,0160	0,0022	0,0166
Abdominal obesity(+)	138	0,1554	0,0001	0,0273	0,0073
Abdominal obesity(-)	10	0,0113	0,0009	0,3763	0,1006
Hypertensive	81	0,0912	0,0064	0,0397	0,1468
Non-hypertensive	67	0,0755	0,0078	0,0480	0,1775
Hypercholesterolemia	60	0,0676	0,0003	0,0364	0,2041
CHOLESTEROLEMIA-Normal	88	0,0991	0,0002	0,0248	0,1392
Hba1c-Unbalanced	29	0,0327	0,3750	0,0035	0,0002
Hba1c-Balanced	119	0,1340	0,0914	0,0009	0,0000
Age groups-23-33 years	8	0,0090	0,0000	0,0000	0,0000
Age groups-34 to 44 years	35	0,0394	0,0000	0,0000	0,0000
Age groups-45 to 55 years	53	0,0597	0,0000	0,0000	0,0000
Age groups-56 to 66 years	41	0,0462	0,0000	0,0000	0,0000
Age groups - over 66	11	0,0124	0,0000	0,0000	0,0000

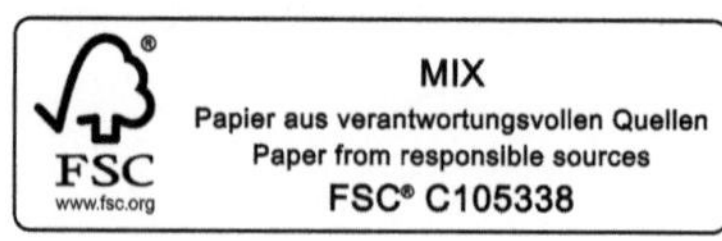

Printed by Books on Demand GmbH, Norderstedt / Germany